KNIFE TO THE HEART

KNIFE
TO THE HEART

The Story of Transplant Surgery

Tony Stark

MACMILLAN

First published 1996 by Macmillan

an imprint of Macmillan General Books
25 Eccleston Place, London SW1W 9NF
and Basingstoke

Associated companies throughout the world

ISBN 0 333 65257 6

1 3 5 7 9 8 6 4 2

A CIP catalogue record for this book is available from
the British Library

Photoset by Parker Typesetting Service, Leicester
Printed and bound in Great Britain by
Mackays of Chatham plc, Chatham, Kent

For Adam and Simon

Contents

List of Illustrations ix

Acknowledgements xiii

Introduction 1

1. Dogs' Legs, Cats' Kidneys and Monkey Glands 7

2. Hard Graft 25

3. The Man with the Golden Hands 55

4. The Knife-edge of Survival 79

5. The Holy Grail 106

6. Dying for an Organ 135

7. A Pig to Save your Bacon 154

8. Brave New Bodies 180

Postscript: The Mystery of Betty's Body 204

Appendix: Transplant Survival Records to end of 1994 209

Notes 215

Bibliography 237

Index 241

List of Illustrations

Alexis Carrel: Nobel-prize-winning surgeon who did some of the earliest transplant experiments. (*Courtesy Rockefeller University*)

Carrel with assistant operating on a dog in 1914. (*Courtesy Rockefeller University*)

John R. Brinkley: the 'quack' doctor who thought he could rejuvenate people by giving them testis transplants. (© *Range*)

Ruth Tucker on the day in July 1950 that she left hospital after her kidney transplant. Shown with her husband and a nurse. (© *Range*)

René Küss: the French surgeon who transplanted a kidney taken from a guillotined prisoner in 1951. (*Courtesy René Küss*)

Jean Hamburger: led the transplant team at the Necker Hospital in Paris in 1952. His first patient given a new kidney lived for just twenty-one days.

David Hume: gave new kidneys to nine patients in Boston between 1951 and 1953. All died early deaths except one who lived for almost six months. (*Courtesy Medical College of Virginia*)

Joseph Murray operating on Richard Herrick – the first successful organ transplant. (*Courtesy Harvard Medical School*)

Richard Herrick seen here with the donor of his transplanted kidney, his identical twin Ronald, and Joseph Murray, the surgeon who gave it to him. They are pictured with two other members of the transplant team that did the world's first successful kidney transplant in 1954. (*Courtesy Harvard Medical School*)

Gladys Lowman: the first patient to be given X-rays to prevent rejection. She died twenty-eight days after her transplant in 1958. (*Courtesy Roy Dalton*)

Peter Medawar. The zoologist who first showed that rejection could be beaten. He was knighted in 1960. (© *Range*)

Roy Calne: the surgeon who helped find the first practical method of preventing rejection in patients. Shown in 1960 with Lollipop, one of his longest-surviving kidney transplant dogs. (*Courtesy Sir Roy Calne*)

Mrs Gen with René Küss. She was the first person to live for more than a year on a kidney transplanted from a completely unrelated donor. (*Courtesy René Küss*)

Yvette Thibault: she's lived longer than anyone else in the world with a kidney transplanted from an unrelated donor. Her operation was in October 1964. (*Courtesy Yvette Thibault*)

Denise Darvall: run over by a car in Cape Town in December 1967. She was the donor in the world's first human heart transplant. (© *Range*)

Louis Washkansky: given a new heart in 1967 in an operation that changed the face of transplant surgery. (© *Range*)

The team that did the world's first human heart transplant in December 1967. Chris Barnard is standing fourth from right in the middle row. (*Courtesy Groote Schur Hospital*)

Louis Washkansky under an oxygen tent shortly after his transplant operation in December 1967. (© *The Cape Argus*)

Jamie Scudero, the second person to be given a new heart. He died six and a half hours after his transplant at Maimonides Medical Centre in New York. (*Courtesy Adrian Kantrowitz*)

Adrian Kantrowitz after his first heart transplant on Jamie Scudero in December 1967. The operation was a failure. (*Courtesy Adrian Kantrowitz*)

Chris and Louwtjie Barnard – in happier days before their separation. (© *Camera Press*)

Chris Barnard besieged by young autograph hunters in Germany in 1968. (© *Range*)

The first picture of Philip Blaiberg after his heart transplant in January 1968. He's shown with Chris Barnard. (© *Range*)

Showing the flag for Britain. The transplant team at the National Heart Hospital in London at a press conference after the first British heart transplant in May 1968. (© *Range*)

Fred West, Britain's first heart transplant patient. He lived just forty-five days after his operation in May 1968. (© *Hulton Deutsch*)

Norman Shumway, the heart surgeon from California, who carried on transplanting hearts when almost everyone else had stopped. (© *Range*)

Everett Thomas, Denton Cooley's first heart transplant patient, shortly after his operation in 1968. (*Courtesy Texas Heart Hospital*)

Denton Cooley: he did more heart transplants in the last eight months of 1968 than anyone else in the world. Most of his patients died early deaths. (*Courtesy Texas Heart Hospital*)

Lorraine Ustipak with John Najarian, the surgeon who bucked the system to save her life. Photographed in 1994. (*Courtesy Lorraine Ustipak*)

William Summerlin – the researcher who was sacked for faking his results. (© *Medical World News*)

Baby Fae: a baboon's heart couldn't save her life. (© *Associated Press*)

Leonard Bailey – life threatened after transplanting a baboon's heart into a baby girl. (© *Associated Press*)

A member of the militant Animal Liberation Front shown after raiding Leonard Bailey's laboratory at Loma Linda University to free experimental animals. (*Courtesy Margo Tannenbaum*)

A monkey's brain removed from its skull and artificially kept alive outside the body by the American neurosurgeon Robert White. (*Courtesy Professor Robert White*)

Robert White pictured with the body of one monkey that has been transplanted on to the head of another. (© *Stern Magazine*)

Another of White's whole body transplants. This one regained consciousness. (*Courtesy Professor Robert White*)

Laura Davies – the little English girl who died after surgeons in Pittsburgh, USA, transplanted six organs into her body. Shown with her mother and father. (© *Press Association*)

Benito Agrelo: the boy who decided to die rather than suffer the side effects of his anti-rejection drugs. (© *Rex Features*)

Betty Baird – the liver transplant patient who threw away all her anti-rejection drugs and lived. (*Courtesy Betty Baird*)

Stephen Hyett: the man whose life was saved by six transplanted organs.

Imutran's genetically engineered pigs. Soon, their organs could be saving people's lives. (*Courtesy Imutran*)

The author and publishers have made every effort to trace the copyright holders of illustrations used in this book. In the event that any have been inadvertently overlooked, please contact the publishers so that the situation can be rectified in future editions.

Acknowledgements

I'd like to thank Jo Rougvie for her invaluable assistance in the preparation of the manuscript. The book was written to a very tight deadline, and would not have been completed on schedule without the well-organized and efficient way in which she conducted the fact-checking research.

Many thanks are also due to George Carey who helped make it possible for me to write this book and whose keen insights have been a great help in clarifying the issues. Unless otherwise stated, the interviews were either conducted by myself or by my colleagues Jenny Barraclough, Ingrid Geser and Richard Pendry who worked with me on the BBC TV series *Knife to the Heart*. I'd like to express my gratitude to them for providing me with such rich material from which to construct the nine chapters in this book.

It is, of course, always helpful to have a fresh eye look over one's work and I am particularly grateful for the views of my editor Georgina Morley and the comments provided by Sir Roy Calne, Ingrid Geser, Chrissy McKean, Tom Starzl and Leslie Wiener – who all kindly agreed to read the manuscript before publication. Their suggestions have significantly improved the narrative.

Finally, I would like to express my thanks to the following either for their assistance with the research or for the uncomplaining way in which they have answered the many questions that I've thrown at them over the past few months: Arasan Aruliah; Leonard Bailey; Habib Beary; Jean Borel; Leslie Brent; Pam Burton; Merrill Chase; Adrian Kantrowitz; Henri Kreis; René Küss; Donald Longmore; Joseph Murray; Stephen Squinto; Paul Terasaki; Andreas Tzakis; David White; Robert White.

TONY STARK

5 December 1995

Introduction

In the early hours of 3 December 1967 a young surgeon walked into an operating theatre in Cape Town, South Africa, carrying a human heart in a metal tray. It was a pivotal moment in the history of spare-part surgery. Until then, transplantation was a therapy that had attracted little attention: doctors only knew how to graft one organ, the kidney and, outside medical circles, people were not desperately interested in the subject. Within a few hours that was going to change. Transplant surgery would capture the imagination of the public in a way that no other surgical procedure has, before or since. The surgeon with the heart in his hands was Dr Christiaan Barnard, and he was on his way to perform the first human heart transplant. Soon the faces of this unknown South African doctor and the businessman whose life he wanted to save would be on the front page of all the world's major newspapers.

The first human heart transplant became as big a story as man's first steps on the moon because, in 1967, many people thought such an operation either could not or should not be performed. After all, wasn't it the heartbeat that told us we were alive? And wasn't the heart also the seat of the soul, the symbol of love and affection? How could we even think about cutting it out and giving it to someone else? It wasn't surprising that the first heart transplant caused such a stir. Even today, if you ask who did the first transplant, you will as likely as not be told about Dr Barnard. That is wrong, of course, but the error is a measure of the impact of the operation he did. In fact, an earlier generation of doctors had struggled for the best part of half a century to persuade the body to accept the gift of life. Without their determination, Barnard would never have been in a position to transplant a human heart.

This book is the story of the painful birth and frequently

controversial first years of a new medical science. Wise minds once dismissed transplant surgery as a scientific impossibility, nothing more than the idle daydreams of sculptors, painters and visionaries. But in little more than a generation, spare-part surgery has become the standard treatment for many incurable diseases. Its pioneers are the doctors and researchers who challenged medical orthodoxy to make a dream come true. One of them is the English transplant surgeon Roy Calne. In 1951, when he was still a medical student at Guy's Hospital in London, Calne was asked to take care of a young man dying of Bright's disease, an incurable illness of the kidneys. Medical science could do nothing for him. In those days, the artificial kidney machine was an experimental treatment that could only prolong life for a matter of days – and, anyway, Guy's Hospital did not have one. Those few brave souls who had attempted to save lives with kidney grafts had not had a single success. The best that doctors could do was to dull the pain with drugs and wait for the patient to die. Roy Calne had the onerous task of tending the teenager as his young life ebbed away.

'His specialist told me he'd be dead in a couple of weeks, so I should try and give him two weeks of reasonable comfort while he was dying,' he explains. 'I knew enough anatomy and physiology to realize the kidneys were the kind of organ that you might graft in much the same way that you'd graft the branches of a fruit tree or a rose bush, so I asked: "Couldn't he have a graft of a kidney?" The consultant physician said: "No. It can't be done." I said: "Why not?" He just said: "It can't be done because it can't be done." One of my friends whispered that I had better not ask any more questions like that if I wanted a job at Guy's!'

Forty-three years later, the now distinguished Sir Roy Calne approached another desperately sick young man who was lying under green drapes and bathed in a pool of light in the centre of an operating theatre at Addenbrooke's Hospital in Cambridge. Sir Roy was about to perform an operation that would have brought his career to an early end, had he suggested it as a student. He was going to transplant six new organs into thirty-two-year-old Stephen Hyett.

For about a year Hyett had watched helplessly as a benign tumour spread through his intestines. As it grew, it blocked arteries, damaged nerves and caused him terrible pain. He had already had three operations: his large bowel had been removed as had half his pancreas and part of his stomach and duodenum. But they failed to prevent the onslaught on his body.

'It was a living death,' Sir Roy explains. 'He was being fed through a vein and was being given vast amounts of pain-killing drugs which dulled his senses. So he wasn't really able to relate in a normal fashion to his family or anyone else. It was a terrible existence. Exactly how long he would have gone on like that I don't know, but I think it was only a matter of months, if that.'

Hyett's only hope was a transplant. Sir Roy had planned to give him a new liver and small intestine. But when he saw how far the illness had spread he realized that only the removal of six of his diseased organs and the insertion of healthy replacements would save the young man's life. In effect, Hyett needed an entirely new digestive system. It's a measure of how far transplant surgery has progressed in the past forty years that any surgeon would consider attempting such a high-risk procedure. But after dedicating nearly four decades of his life to transplant surgery, Sir Roy Calne felt sufficiently confident of his abilities and those of the team he had trained to push the boundaries of medical science one step further into the unknown.

It took eight hours to remove Hyett's liver, stomach, duodenum, pancreas, small bowel and one of his kidneys. A further five hours were needed to sew in the six replacements. Today, nearly two years after his life-saving operation, the patient is back at home near Cambridge, enjoying the life that he so nearly lost.

'I don't need to take any pain-killing drugs at all now,' says Hyett. 'I couldn't eat before. Now I can eat like a normal person . . . I go out shopping with my wife, which was impossible before and I can play with my children. It's a vast improvement. I still really haven't got over what they've done to me.'

Transplant surgery is young enough for many of its pioneering surgeons, physicians and medical researchers to be alive today. Their struggles, their victories and defeats, are mostly told first-hand. But there is a different kind of pioneer to whom transplantation owes an incalculable debt: those desperately ill patients who agreed to co-operate with untried and unproved treatments and who frequently lost their lives in the process. Endless failures dogged the steps of the early transplanters and these pages belong as much to those who suffered early deaths as they do to the determined surgeons who wielded the knife. Without their courage there would be no transplant surgery.

The problem that faced the first transplant surgeons, and which continues to plague spare-part surgery, is simple to describe but almost impossible to overcome: the body cannot tell the difference between a grafted organ and a dangerous bacterium or virus. A transplant is seen as a foreign invader that must be destroyed as rapidly and effectively as any other infectious bug. The human immune system is very good at its job but it is blind to the life-saving benefits of a graft and works ceaselessly to bring about the patient's and, ultimately, its own downfall. It took surgeons decades to find a way of preventing 'rejection', the body's attempt to rid itself of a transplant. And when the once-impregnable fortress of the immune system was finally breached, there was a high price to pay. Patients faced new terrors brought on by the drugs, like steroids, that were keeping them alive. Doctors and their transplanted patients walked a fine line: too low a dose of drugs and the transplant ceased to function. Too high, and they were poisoned or their immune systems became so weak that they died of other, opportunistic infections. It was a delicate balancing act.

Today there are better treatments to prevent rejection – as Stephen Hyett's life-saving operation so dramatically demonstrates. There are many other examples. People who a decade or two ago would have faced certain death from kidney, heart or liver failure are today living with other people's organs inside them. Many gain an extra five years of life. Some are still alive at ten, twenty and even thirty years later. As surgical skills and the ability to prevent the body destroying a grafted organ have improved, so the range of life-saving transplants has increased. Even once-incurable inherited illnesses are beginning to fall to the onward march of spare-part surgery. New lungs can end the suffocating misery of cystic fibrosis. Pancreatic cell transplants are being hailed as a possible cure for Parkinson's disease. Diabetes is under attack by the transplanters. They are even beginning to tackle some cancers, like leukaemia.

But every step forward has been accompanied by a host of daunting ethical dilemmas. Was it right, many wondered in the early days, to take a kidney out of one person to save the life of another? Wouldn't such an operation be risking the donor's health – and didn't this break the most basic tenet of the medical profession: the instruction to do no harm? This question was the source of endless arguments and anxiety. There were others. After Barnard did his transplant, there was heated debate about the rights and wrongs of removing a human heart while it was still beating from the body. This was the only way of making heart transplantation a reality, but many thought it amounted to murder. Was there, as the surgeons argued, a more sensible way of defining death, one that would permit them to retrieve hearts fresh enough to continue beating in another body? Or were such suggestions an affront to civilized standards? These were far from merely academic questions: surgeons were taken to court and charged with killing their patients before this vexed issue was resolved.

Today different issues dog the footsteps of transplant surgeons but the dilemmas have more than kept pace with the new technology. Doctors might now have the drugs to keep their transplanted patients alive, but they haven't got anything like enough organs. With many terminally ill people pleading for every transplantable liver, lung, heart and kidney how do you decide who is the most deserving? Reluctant doctors are forced to play God – giving life to the lucky few, leaving the rest to queue up for organs that sometimes never arrive. More and more patients are dying on waiting lists. None of the solutions offered so far has solved the problem and one or two have been met with howls of protest. The latest attempt is every bit as controversial as all the rest. Some scientists have come to the conclusion that there will never be enough human organs to supply all those in need.

But there are plenty of animals and if their organs could be used to fill the gap, they would have the problem licked. The problem is, of course, that nothing raises the public's hackles more than the sight of scientists experimenting on animals. Their use by transplant surgeons has already aroused angry protests. One grafted a baboon's heart into a baby and had to wear a flak jacket for several months after the operation. Another's home was vandalized for genetically engineering pigs to make their organs compatible with the human body.

Despite the controversies, organ grafting has earned its place as the medical miracle of the century. It has opened surgical doors that would have seemed inconceivable a bare fifty years ago. It has given birth to the study of immunology, an entirely new discipline that has contributed to many different fields of medicine. And the next fifty years will undoubtedly bring similar marvels. Will there come a day when changing your heart or your lungs becomes as simple as changing the carburettor in a car? Will amputees ever benefit from limb transplants? And what about the human brain: is it technically possible to transplant this most complicated of organs? Is it morally permissible? Robert White, an American neurosurgeon, has already done it and is in no doubt that the answer to both these questions is yes. In the 1970s and 1980s, White pioneered operations in Cleveland, Ohio, that some describe as repugnant and unethical. He has transplanted monkey heads onto other monkeys' bodies. His ambition is to become the first surgeon in the world to transplant a human body onto a human head.

'If you will only look at history and where we have come in the past forty years, there's no question that it is possible and that soon after the turn of the century it will be done,' says White.

But should it be done? There's little doubt that whatever wonders spare-part surgery's creative minds conjure up in the future, the ethical questions they raise will more than keep pace with the developing technology.

1

Dogs' Legs, Cats' Kidneys and Monkey Glands

In 1894 France was engulfed in a wave of political ferment. It was a time of bombings, protests and turmoil. There were bloody clashes between police and disgruntled workers, angered by the poverty and inequality in their society. The anarchist flag was flying high. In the midst of all this chaos, Santo Caserio, a twenty-year-old baker's assistant, abruptly quit his job in the town of Cette. He took his meagre wages to a cutlery shop where he bought an ornate knife with a six-inch blade before jumping on the next train to the city of Lyon. Caserio was an anarchist with vengeance on his mind. He had set off to murder Sadi Carnot, the President of the French Republic, in revenge for his refusal to reprieve a comrade condemned to the guillotine for throwing a bomb. Caserio wanted to transform the destiny of France. Little did he realize that his knife would be the catalyst for the birth of transplant surgery. For in Lyon there lived another young man with a passion for knives: Alexis Carrel, a twenty-one-year-old doctor at the Red Cross Hospital, who would soon be recognized as one of the most innovative surgeons of his generation. Caserio's impulsive action and the direction of Carrel's professional life became inextricably intertwined.

Once in Lyon, the anarchist wrapped his weapon in a copy of *La Républicain*, and mingled with the crowd waiting for the President. Despite the dissent, Carnot was a popular man: thousands of cheering people were on the streets and the threat of anarchist violence did not stop him from pressing the flesh. He told the police to allow people to approach his open carriage. It was a fatal decision. As Carnot drove into sight, the baker's assistant seized his chance. Pushing several spectators aside, he unsheathed his knife and ran towards the carriage. He grabbed the side of the vehicle with his left hand and lunged forward, pushing the blade deep into Carnot's stomach. The ornate knife punctured the President's liver and severed his portal vein, one of the major blood vessels in the body. The crowds cheered as Carnot was driven off at high speed. Most were unaware that their President's life-blood was ebbing away inside the carriage.

Six doctors fought to save his life, but in the 1890s, the severing of a major artery or vein often led to the loss of a limb (if you were lucky) or the loss of your life (if you weren't). Although they could join tissues like the skin, surgeons were unable to sew blood vessels – veins and arteries – together with any measure of success. The attempt to do so invariably damaged the inner wall, producing blood clots which blocked the vessel, rendering it useless. Carnot was unlucky: a plumbing problem cost him his life. It was a tragedy but an unavoidable one, according to most nineteenth-century surgeons.

That wasn't the view of young Alexis Carrel. Carnot's assassination made a big impression on the young doctor. He insisted that the President's life should have been saved, and told friends and superiors at the hospital that he found it hard to believe that surgeons had not yet perfected the art of anastomosis – the technical term for the sewing together of blood vessels.

Carrel cut a distinctive figure at the Red Cross Hospital. A generous inheritance from his grandparents allowed him to dress with Parisian elegance. He wore thick *pince-nez* glasses to correct myopia and only when these were removed was it possible to see his piercing eyes: one brown and the other blue. Those who knew him say he was an intense, distant and conceited man with a highly original, stimulating mind. But he could also be distracted and absent-minded, and was sometimes seen to drive on the pavement or the wrong way up one-way streets.

Carrel was never slow to offer his opinions and said what he felt with a refreshing but at times naïve abandon. In later years, his support for the gassing of criminals, his desire to prevent the 'unintelligent' from having the vote and his belief in the inequality of the sexes brought considerable criticism. But his scientific ideas were usually sound and frequently aired. Over time the stabbing of President Carnot faded from public memory, but it was never far from Carrel's thoughts: he was convinced that there must be a safe method of rejoining blood vessels. Four years after the assassination, he left the daily grind of hospital work to take up a lecturing post in the faculty of medicine at the University of Lyon. It was here that he began the search for a solution and so took the first steps on a path that eventually made him the true father of transplant surgery.

Most forms of surgery rely on the ability to rejoin blood vessels, but the transplantation of organs depends entirely on this technique. The only way a surgeon can restore the circulation to a transplant is by joining the organ's blood vessels to those in the recipient. It is routine work today and the diagrams in biology books make it look easy: one expertly drawn and perfectly circular artery is placed next to another, the ends meet and they are stitched together. On the operating table, of course, things are different: those nice round tubes have become flat and flaccid, bearing as little similarity to the text-book diagrams as a chewed drinking straw does to its unsucked equivalent. Considerable dexterity is needed to rejoin blood vessels, particularly the small ones – and when it came to sewing, Alexis Carrel was a perfectionist. He would spend hours practising, stitching together pieces of paper until he could join them firmly without puncturing a hole in either one. He even took lessons in embroidery to hone his skills, putting up with the taunts of colleagues with little complaint. By the time he was thirty, Carrel's sewing skill could put that of most professional seamstresses to shame. But manual dexterity was only part of the answer: he also needed a way to turn back those flaccid veins and arteries into tubes before he could sew them together. The elegant technique he devised is still used, with only minor modifications, today. He sewed three equally spaced stitches around the circumference of each of the cut ends of the blood vessels that he wished to join together. By pulling on all three stitches at once, the vessel opened up, its end shaped like a triangle, making the task of joining one end to the other relatively easy. Carrel used very fine thread and sharp, round needles coated with Vaseline to seal the holes in the vessels as soon as they were made, thereby preventing blood from coming into contact with the damaged vessel. At the turn of the century, this was revolutionary and opened up an entirely new field of life-saving surgery.

It also aroused Carrel's interest in transplantation: he began to wonder if his new technique could be used to repair damaged blood vessels. He experimented on dogs, joining arteries to veins or patching them with veins, and demonstrated that such grafts were a practical method of saving lives. It took forty years for his technique to find its way into clinical practice but it is now a mainstay of vascular surgery.

Carrel also believed his technique could be used to rejoin an amputated limb. To prove this, he cut off and then replaced the hind leg of a dog, rejoining its blood vessels and quickly sewing it back in place. All went well until, unnoticed by the surgeon, the plaster covering the leg of the unfortunate animal slipped, allowing the dog to urinate into the wound, which promptly went septic. The leg did not survive – and neither did the dog. But Carrel's technique was used by surgeons at the Massachusetts General Hospital in 1962 when they rejoined the arm of a twelve-year-old boy who had been run over by a train – the first time a human limb had been successfully reattached to its owner.[1]

Alexis Carrel's irrepressible medical curiosity pushed him deeper and deeper into the transplant world. Was it possible, he wondered, for an animal to survive after the removal and replacement of one of its organs? He wasn't the first to attempt to answer this question,[2] but his meticulous scientific approach and keen powers of observation identified for the first time what could and – importantly – what could not be done. His first transplants took place at the University of Lyon. He chose the kidney for his experiments, because it was easy to remove, had a simple blood supply and an obvious, measurable function. In 1902 he began a series of transplants, removing the right kidney from a dog and re-implanting it into the neck of the same animal, where it was relatively easy to inspect. The end of the ureter (the tube that normally carries urine from the kidney to the bladder) was stitched to a small opening in the skin next to the dog's breast bone. The neck kidneys worked for a while but infection brought these experiments to a premature end: the dogs died of gangrene. By 1907 Carrel had emigrated to America and was working at the prestigious Rockefeller Institute in New York. It was here that he began a new series of transplants that brought him notoriety and, eventually, a Nobel Prize. His operating room was on the top floor of the building with east-facing windows that flooded it with bright sunlight. In those days surgeons generally wore white, but sunlight reflects off white and strains the eyes so Carrel insisted all his staff wear special clothing. Merrill Chase is one of the few people alive who still remembers Alexis Carrel: he worked with him at the Rockefeller Institute in the 1930s and recalls the arcane air of mystery that the clothing gave to his work. 'He dressed all in black. All of his technicians wore black. The girls only had space in their black masks – four inches across by two and a half – so that you could see their eyes. Their hands were tucked inside their black gowns and they stood against the background waiting for the master to need something.'

To minimize the risk of infection, Carrel abandoned the neck as a home for his transplanted kidneys and instead replaced his grafted organs in the abdominal cavity where they belonged. He worked with both dogs and cats, this time removing both kidneys before performing the transplant: either putting back the kidneys into the same animal or transplanting them into a different one. 'The efficiency of the transplanted organ,' wrote Carrel, 'would be absolutely demonstrated if the host lived in good health and secreted normal urine.'[3]

The results were clear cut: animals that were grafted with their own kidneys survived to live normal lives; those given the kidneys of another animal invariably died. The transplanted organs worked for a few days or weeks after the operations, but then mysteriously ceased to function. Carrel didn't know it but he had discovered 'rejection', one of the most fundamental of evolutionary principles: the process by which an organism seeks out and destroys anything foreign in its system. Rejection doomed all organ grafts between different animals in the first half of the

twentieth century. 'I have never found positive results to continue
after a few months,' Carrel wrote in 1914. 'The biological side of
the question has to be investigated very much more and we must
find out by what means to prevent the reaction of the organism
against a new organ.'[4]

If Carrel was upset at his inability to keep his transplanted
animals alive, the animal rights lobby was incensed. One irate
anti-vivisectionist resorted to irony: 'The kidneys of one set of
cats and dogs had been cut out and transplanted in other cats and
dogs,' he wrote indignantly. 'And one dog, apparently by way of
diversion, had, according to the report, been supplied with
kidneys which had been located in its neck instead of in the loins
. . . The fact is noted that the animals were able to display all the
natural propensities of their kind – the cats to spit and the dogs to
growl. This is not surprising.'[5]

But there was anger too: 'The doctors who do this sort of
thing,' complained another animal lover, 'are not only out of jail
but are boasting of their prowess. What would a civilized parent
do to his boy if he caught him in such practices?' A third
castigated Carrel as a 'monster and a demon who should be
condemned to the electric chair'.[6] There was even a death threat:
'Remember,' wrote a poetic 'admirer' in a hand-written note
dropped through Carrel's letterbox, 'when death is drawing near
and your heart sinks in fear, you are going to reap what you have
sown. No mercy.'[7] Animal rights activists were a thorn in Carrel's
side and have continued to dog the footsteps of transplant surgery
ever since.

Outside their intense ranks, however, there was considerable
enthusiasm for his pioneering transplant work. Carrel once even
had to turn away a patient who asked the by then famous surgeon
to stitch back a severed arm. History does not record the reason
for the refusal but perhaps Carrel decided he was not ready to
expand his repertoire of transplant techniques. The request might
have rekindled his interest in limb grafts, though, because in 1908
he began an extensive series of experimental transplants in which
he swapped legs between dogs in his laboratory in the Rockefeller
Institute. One visitor was greeted with the strange sight of a black

fox terrier walking around with a white foreleg, and a yellow animal 'hopping along gaily',[8] as he put it, also with a white leg. This visitor was impressed with the health and vitality of the new limbs – he saw the dogs just six days after they were transplanted. Had he returned to the laboratory a few days later, he would have seen the skin peeling from the grafted limbs as they swelled and turned blue. The mysterious 'biological force' proved as unremittingly destructive with Carrel's leg transplants as it had been with his kidneys.

In the first ten years of this century Carrel also tried grafting the thyroid gland, the ovaries, and even a dog's heart, which beat for a short time, but the message from these experiments was clear and unambiguous. With the correct surgical techniques, organs could be removed and retransplanted to the same animal with no ill effects; animals given a foreign organ, however, invariably died within a few weeks of their operation.

In 1914 Alexis Carrel received the ultimate scientific accolade when he was awarded the Nobel Prize in Medicine for his pioneering surgical and transplant work. 'Sir, you have accomplished great things,' read the citation. 'You have invented a new method of suturing[9] blood vessels! . . . You have succeeded in the most daring and extremely difficult operations . . .'[10]

Carrel's work had helped to transform organ transplantation from an idle dream into a distinct possibility. Although he never found an answer to rejection – and urged caution on anyone thinking of grafting organs from one animal to another – transplantation captured the public imagination. People wanted to believe it could work – so strongly that, by the 1920s, Carrel's words of warning were drowned in a wave of what can only be described as transplant fever or, perhaps more appropriately, glandular fever. One organ was the focus of all the fuss: the male testis gland, long believed to be linked to sexual vigour and longevity but now elevated by a potent combination of surgical skill, mythology and greed into an icon.

For centuries people had believed in the aphrodisiac and rejuvenating powers of the testis. It was a myth, but the Greeks used it and so did the Romans: the Emperor Caligula is said to have swallowed extracts of wolf testes in his debauched binges although their most marked effect would have been to leave a bad taste in his mouth. The myth ran deep. In 1889 Charles Edouard Brown-Séquard, a distinguished seventy-two-year-old French physiologist who was suffering the debilitating effects of ageing, announced that he had successfully reversed his decline with injections of testis extract. 'Everything I had not been able to do or had done badly for several years on account of my advanced age I am today able to perform most admirably,' he told a stunned audience at the Société de Biologie in Paris.

No controlled scientific experiments existed to test such wild claims, but at the end of the nineteenth century medical researchers tried to isolate extracts of the mysterious rejuvenating substance from the testis. When they failed, some turned to grafting the gland itself, stitching slices of testicle into the scrotum in the belief that such treatment would reverse ageing or increase sexual virility. The grafts couldn't have done this even if they had survived because testosterone, the hormone produced by the testis, has none of the powers claimed by its supporters.[11] But they didn't know this at the end of the nineteenth century. They also didn't know that the gland grafts would all have been destroyed in a matter of days, rejected by the same mysterious biological force that baffled Carrel, but many were taken in by a gullible and greedy few who were more than happy to prey on people's naïveté.

John R. Brinkley was one of them. He called himself a doctor; in fact, he was a quack. His university degree was fraudulent and the rest of his medical education was clouded in obscurity. But 'Dr' Brinkley was no fool. He had an excellent knowledge of anatomy and surgical technique, and from 1917 ran a private medical practice in the sleepy town of Milford, a small Mid-Western town in Kansas. Brinkley's career as a transplant surgeon began when a patient asked if he could be cured of his impotence by a testis transplant. Brinkley agreed to try, so long as the patient would supply the testis. He arrived for his transplant holding a goat.

'To me the results were amazing and startling because I

expected bad results and disastrous results and instead of that happy results were obtained,' Brinkley later explained. 'The man claimed he had been sexually dead for sixteen years. His wife verified that statement. A year later I delivered his wife of a fine baby boy.'[12]

The miracle baby was appropriately named Billy, and Brinkley never looked back. He offered to rejuvenate people with goat testis transplants, and coined the catchy slogan 'You are only as old as your glands'. He was soon raking in the cash. Brinkley performed a range of operations, the most expensive costing $750, which was a small fortune at the time. By the mid 1920s, he had built a well-equipped fifty-bed hospital in Milford and was shipping in twenty-five goats a week. Patients recovering from their operations could hear them bleating in an open pen two blocks away from the hospital. If the noise got too much to bear, the thoughtful Dr Brinkley provided each bed with a pair of earphones so that patients could tune into KFKB, Kansas First Kansas Best, Brinkley's own 1000-watt radio station. KFKB opened in 1923 when broadcasting was new and decent equipment hard to get. It was the most powerful in America and, needless to say, Brinkley used it to spread the good word. The recurrent theme of his nightly medical broadcasts was the need for older men to restore their virility by having a goat-gland transplant. At the height of his success, John R. Brinkley received three thousand letters a day from people seeking medical advice. It wasn't surprising that he became exceptionally wealthy, eventually owning several homes, cars, a yacht and two aeroplanes.

What was surprising, though, was the wide-ranging support for gland grafting among the medical profession. In the 1920s, Brinkley was by no means alone in his mistaken belief in the efficacy of the treatment he was offering. With no rigorous examination of the anecdotal claims of success, many respectable doctors were convinced that the elixir of youth lay hidden inside the humble testicle, which helped create the climate in which Brinkley could amass such a fortune. He would never have succeeded had he been the only practitioner in the field.

Dr Leo Stanley, the medical officer of San Quentin Prison in

California, was certainly no quack, but he was a gland grafter, using the testicles of freshly executed prisoners to 'rejuvenate' inmates suffering from premature ageing (a complaint exacerbated, perhaps, by the harsh regime in the jail). He did thirty such operations. George Frank Lydston, a respectable surgeon and professor of genito-urinary surgery and venereal disease in Chicago, was also doing testis transplants. He, too, used human testicles and claimed beneficial effects on patients suffering from various degenerative diseases. Lydston even grafted one onto himself, and to prove it once dropped his trousers in front of Max Thorek, another gland grafter. He 'astonished his colleague by showing him what he said was the transplanted testicle in place close to his own testicles,' says the author, David Hamilton. 'Lydston told Thorek that the transplant had invigorated him greatly.'[13] Unfortunately, the rejuvenation claimed by Lydston was entirely psychological. He died three years later of pneumonia.

'Glandular' fever was not solely an American phenomenon. At least three surgeons were doing it in London; a Russian surgeon had a brief flirtation with the testis; two Italian doctors leapt on the bandwagon. But the most prolific and well known of all the 'respectable' gland grafters was the flamboyant Paris surgeon Sergei Voronoff. Voronoff was a Russian *émigré* who became a French citizen in 1895. His early medical career was conventional: he wrote books about surgery and gynaecology; he established a nurses' training college; he started a medical magazine and spent some time in Egypt as the personal physician of Khedive Abbas II, the country's ruler. When he reached his mid forties Voronoff became interested in tissue transplantation and rapidly became the most famous of all the gland grafters. He saw himself as a scientist, giving papers on his work at international conferences and publishing long accounts of the results of his operations and the theory of gland grafting. In one, he explained why he had chosen to use monkey testicles.

I use the glands of monkeys . . . because the securing of human glands presents serious obstacles and because the glands of monkeys . . . are the only ones that can furnish grafts which will find, among human tissues, the same conditions of life that they had originally. To use the glands of other animals is to ignore completely the laws of biology: they could never be, in the human organism, anything but foreign bodies.[14]

Voronoff was wrong, of course. Monkey glands were rejected like any other foreign object placed in the human body. This would not have been obvious to the surgeon as the dead graft would remain in place next to the patient's own testicle, an inert lump, its cellular structure destroyed and replaced by cells from the body. But Voronoff's pseudo-scientific words had two effects: they helped give testis transplants the veneer of respectability and they further stoked the flames of 'glandular' fever. He once claimed that he could 'put back human ageing by twenty to thirty years'.[15] He even told the delegates at one scientific conference that the beneficial effects of gland grafting could be passed on to the next generation.[16] At another, he flirted with the then increasingly popular eugenics movement and announced that gland grafting early in life could increase the mental and physical powers of gifted children. 'I call for children of genius,' he announced. 'Give me such children and I will create a new super-race of men of genius.'[17]

At the height of his gland-grafting days, Voronoff imported hundreds of baboons from Africa. He kept them in a large *palazzo* on the Italian Riviera, employing a circus animal-keeper to care for them. By 1926 he had done about a thousand grafts, charging as much as £1,000 for each transplant. But Voronoff's motive in making such extravagant claims for testis transplants was not financial: he was already wealthy with an inherited income of more than £200,000 a year. Rather, he had a sincere but misplaced belief in his rejuvenation treatment and used it to secure himself a place in history. He became a celebrity who always provided good copy for the popular and specialist press. In the mid 1920s the question wasn't whether testis transplants could rejuvenate, but how far the technique would eventually be taken. 'Even death, save by accident, may become unknown,' read one eulogistic article in the *Scientific American* in 1924, 'if the daring experiments of Dr Sergei Voronoff, brilliant French surgeon, continue to produce results such as have startled the world.'[18]

Voronoff was honoured with several awards, among them the French Legion of Honour and the Spanish Order of Elizabeth. He was asked to write an entry for the 1926 edition of the *Encyclopaedia Britannica*. Dozens of surgeons visited him to learn about his methods. But it was an obscure Hungarian insurance company that must have given him the most satisfaction when, in 1927, they refused to pay a pension to one of his gland-grafted patients. The company reneged on the contract because they believed the man really was younger than his chronological age. What the patient felt about the refusal is quite another matter, of course.

Sergei Voronoff achieved immortality – but not the kind he would have wanted. The surgeon's downfall began in 1929 with the discovery of testosterone, the hormone produced by the testis. Its function was quickly isolated: castrated rats, for example, would regain some of their male characteristics after treatment with the substance, but laboratory tests proved conclusively that testosterone could not reverse ageing or increase sexual potency. In the 1930s Voronoff's work came increasingly under attack from medical researchers who tried – and failed – to reproduce his results in animals. They had been more rigorous in their scientific approach than had Voronoff, and the death-knell was sounding on the era of the testis transplant. The technique was soon discredited and several of its strongest supporters in the 1920s did their best to forget they had had anything to do with it: 'Dr Stanley retired from San Quentin in 1954 and the booklet put together to mark this occasion omits his pioneering gland-grafting work,' says David Hamilton. 'Even the obituaries which followed the death of Max Thorek in 1960 at the age of eighty, fail to record his ten-year obsession with testis transplantation.'[19] And Kenneth Walker, an English surgeon who announced his own limited 'success' with testis transplants in the 1920s was singing a different tune thirty years later. In a book published in

1952 he said Voronoff's transplants were 'no better than the methods of witches and magicians'.[20]

Testis transplants might have fallen out of fashion but Voronoff wasn't unduly put off by the critics. Doggedly, he continued to champion a lost cause, even publishing a book in 1943 containing 'before' and 'after' pictures in defence of his rejuvenation work. He died after a fall in 1951. Few noted the event. 'The *New York Times*, unaware of their earlier interest in him, not only misspelt his name but concluded that "few took his claims seriously," '[21] says David Hamilton.

A worse fate befell Dr John R. Brinkley. In 1929, the Kansas Board of Medical Registration and Examination banned him from practising medicine in the state after proving that his medical qualifications were fraudulent. He moved to Texas where, nine years later, he sued the editor of *Hygeia* (the journal of the American Medical Association) for calling him a 'quack'. Brinkley lost the action, and with it, his licence to practise medicine in Texas too. Not long after this he declared himself bankrupt.

If they achieved nothing else, the gland grafters whetted the public's appetite for transplantation, and while some members of the medical profession flirted with an unattainable fantasy, others had been making serious attempts to turn the dream into a reality. One was Dr Mathieu Jaboulay, the professor of clinical surgery at the Faculty of Medicine in Lyon, the same city that had nurtured the young Alexis Carrel. Like Carrel, Jaboulay was determined to keep his country in the forefront of medical research. In January 1906 he became the first surgeon to try to save the life of a patient with an organ graft when he transplanted a kidney into a forty-eight-year-old woman suffering from a chronic disease of her own kidneys. The patient's eyesight and hearing were failing. She had severe hypertension. Her life was ebbing away and Jaboulay had nothing else to offer her. He took a leap into the unknown by removing a kidney from a pig and joining it to the blood vessels of his patient's left arm. Jaboulay hoped the new organ might clear her blood of the waste products that were slowly poisoning her. It is probably just as well that he knew nothing of the biological problems of such a transplant, because organs grafted between such distantly related species as the pig and a human are subject to a much fiercer form of rejection than are organs transplanted among the same species. This is known as hyperacute rejection and it may be so severe that a transplant is destroyed within hours. Had Jaboulay realized how high the stakes were he would not, perhaps, have taken the risk. In fact, his pig's kidney survived for two days, produced urine and cleaned waste products from his patient's blood. On the third day it stopped abruptly. When Jaboulay removed the bandage, it showed all the classic signs of hyperacute rejection. 'The exposed surface of the kidney was blue, blackish in places and its temperature only 32 degrees,' he explained that year in a French medical journal. 'Since thrombosis was evident, the kidney was removed . . .'[22]

Jaboulay tried again in April the same year, this time using a goat's kidney, but with no greater success. Three days after the operation, it, too, had to be removed. He abandoned transplant operations after that.

The baton then passed to Ernest Unger, a Jewish surgeon who ran a private clinic in Berlin. 'Can we,' he wondered, 'transplant new, functional kidneys into a person with diseased kidneys, a person who is doomed because he no longer possesses functioning kidneys? Can we implant in some way or other one or two new kidneys, and where do we obtain the kidneys?'[23]

He answered the last of these questions by turning to the Borneo Macaque monkey. He would have preferred to use human kidneys but decided that the practical and ethical problems were too many to overcome. So, in 1909, when a twenty-one-year-old seamstress in the last stages of kidney failure was brought to his clinic, he transplanted both kidneys from a Macaque monkey into the woman's left leg. Her last hours were spent lying on her back with her leg suspended in the air. She died thirty-two hours after the operation, another victim of the seemingly irresistible force of rejection. Unger's conclusions made depressing reading: 'Up to now there has never been any conclusive proof that foreign tissue is accepted in the body of the host,' he wrote. 'Thus our work provides no conclusive results: it simply provides us with a series of new tasks, and the work of many people will be required to shed light on this difficult problem.'[24]

After these dismal failures, few were prepared to risk reputations and careers by treading in these uncharted waters. Over the next thirty years only two surgeons were game enough to try it. In 1923 Harold Neuhof, an American, transplanted a kidney from a lamb into a human patient. It produced a minute amount of urine – but the patient died nine days later. 'A definite conclusion cannot be drawn as to whether or not the transplant functioned as such at any time,' Neuhof concluded.[25] In 1936, the same year that Nazi persecution forced Unger to close his clinic in Berlin, a Soviet surgeon also tried to make the transplant dream come true. Yu Yu Voronoy had read about Jaboulay's and Unger's operations and concluded that the use of animal organs was a waste of time. 'Transplantation of primate organs [Unger] and, above all, of domestic animals such as the goat and pig [Jaboulay] have failed utterly,' he wrote. 'The only source of grafts is the cadaver since the donor does not suffer a loss . . .'[26] Voronoy wanted to use a human kidney but ethical qualms forced him to reject the idea of live organ donation – that battle would not be fought for another two decades. Instead the Soviet surgeon decided to use the next best thing: a human kidney taken from a dead body. In 1936 a twenty-six-year-old woman was rushed to the All-Ukrainian Institute of Surgery and Emergency Blood Transfusion suffering from poisoning. She had tried to commit suicide by swallowing mercuric chloride, a popular household disinfectant. Under the strain of the toxic chemical, her kidneys had stopped working and she was hovering at death's door. To save her life, Voronoy took a kidney from a sixty-year-old man who had just died in the hospital and transplanted it into her body, joining it to the blood vessels in her thigh. In so doing he became the first surgeon to transplant a human organ. The new kidney produced urine for two days, then failed.[27] The woman died a short time later. Yet Voronoy saw hope where others might have seen only despair: 'We firmly believe in the applicability of the method as a therapeutic procedure, once the technical details are better understood, above all the immunologic reactions between the tissue and the serum of the donor and recipients.'[28]

By the end of the 1930s, though, the transplant record was a bleak one, and the next ten years saw only one other, short-lived effort to force the human body to accept the gift of life.[29] Long-term success continued to elude the transplanters until, at the start of the Second World War, the nature of the beast that had destroyed every transplant between different individuals began at last to reveal itself. This was a vital step, for without an understanding of the body's unremitting ability to destroy grafted organs there could be no substantial attempt to combat it.

The man who made the breakthrough was Peter Medawar, a young research scientist working at the Zoology Department of Oxford University. It was during the mid 1940s that fate stepped in to guide Medawar to his discovery. One summer's afternoon he was sunbathing in his garden with his wife and their eldest daughter when they heard the drone of an aeroplane. They looked up to see a bomber flying low over the rooftops straight towards their home. Thinking this was a daylight attack by the Luftwaffe, the Medawars raced for safety. They didn't realize that the plane was an RAF bomber in serious trouble. 'My wife quickly picked up our daughter and bundled her into our air-raid shelter,' Medawar recollects. 'The bomber crashed into the garden of a house about two hundred yards away and immediately exploded with a fearful WHUMP!'[30]

Like the assassination of President Carnot half a century earlier, it was one of those moments in history when personal tragedy and individual destiny coincide. One man survived the crash: a young member of the plane's crew, who was rushed to Oxford's Radcliffe Infirmary with terrible injuries – over 60 per cent of his skin had been destroyed by third-degree burns. The doctors didn't know what to do for him, but one, Dr John Barnes, knew that Medawar had been researching the treatment of severe burns. He asked the young scientist to take a look at his patient.

Medawar was stumped. He knew that rejection would prevent him from transplanting the airman with skin taken from someone else, and there wasn't enough of his own undamaged skin to use for grafting. Instead he tried tissue-culturing small bits of the man's surviving skin, speeding up their growth and then re-transplanting them over damaged areas of his body. The technique failed and, with no other options, Medawar was forced to look again at the problem of rejection. 'I guessed,' he explained, 'that if one could use what were then known as "homografts" – that is to say grafts transplanted from relatives or from other voluntary donors – the treatment of war wounds would be transformed.'[31]

This became Medawar's life's work. Within ten years his pioneering research had become the cornerstone of transplantation. It gave rise to an entirely new field of science and earned him the highest of honours: a knighthood and a Nobel prize. If Alexis Carrel provided the practical skills that made organ grafts a reality, Peter Medawar furnished the theoretical understanding.

The Medical Research Council was only too happy to give the zoologist a grant to investigate skin grafting – after all, this was wartime and there was a desperate need for new treatments to help the increasing numbers of burn victims. So Medawar moved to Glasgow, spending his nights in a hotel in the Colebrook district and his days at the burns unit of Glasgow Royal Infirmary with Tom Gibson, a Scottish surgeon. Working with badly burned patients, Medawar made the first of two discoveries that breathed new life into the almost moribund world of transplant surgery. He grafted small patches of skin[32] taken from a volunteer donor on to the body of an epileptic woman who had been badly burned when she fell against a gas fire. At the same time he transplanted patches taken from the woman herself. For a few days there was little to choose between the two sets of grafts – but it soon became clear that the donor's skin was being rejected while her own grafted skin survived. That was only to be expected. But then Medawar took a second set of skin patches from the same volunteer donor and grafted them on to the woman. What happened next transformed our understanding of the process of rejection: the new grafts were destroyed much more rapidly than the first. This time there was no 'period of grace', in which the body temporarily tolerated the transplanted skin. It had learnt to recognize the graft as foreign and reacted against it immediately. This was a fundamental observation: rejection was not, as everyone then thought, an unchangeable, genetically determined process. It was acquired in much the same way as the body learns to recognize and destroy bacteria and viruses. Medawar's report of this work[33] laid the foundation stone of the science of immunology, which today occupies the efforts of thousands of researchers all over the world. It was also the first of two theoretical building blocks that eventually gave fresh hope to surgeons who wanted to turn transplant surgery into a life-saving reality. But ten years were to pass before Medawar proved that, in the laboratory at least, rejection could be overcome. The 1950s were a decade in which transplant surgery suffered several false dawns.

2

Hard Graft

Fate had dealt Ruth Tucker's family in Chicago the unkindest of hands. For several decades, a minute error in the genetic code had lain dormant inside the Tuckers' bodies. It was a time bomb with a long fuse, quietly ticking away the years until the day it unleashed a slow and painful death on its unfortunate owner. When they were in their thirties or forties, Ruth Tucker's mother, sister and uncle all died of polycystic kidney disease. Her cousin was suffering from it and now Ruth, a telephonist at the Sears and Roebuck store in Chicago, knew her days were numbered. She had tender swellings on either side of her stomach; she suffered terrible back pains, was constantly having to urinate and continually fell ill with a variety of urinary-tract infections. In desperation, her doctor had referred her to Dr Richard H. Lawler, a surgeon working at Loyola University's Stritch School of Medicine with an interest in transplantation. The tests he performed offered Ruth little hope of recovery; her left kidney had failed completely; her right one was down to only 10 per cent of its normal function. It was 1950, Ruth was forty-four and no longer expected to reach forty-five. Lawler had done some experimental kidney grafts on dogs with little success; rejection had destroyed all the transplanted organs within two weeks. But Ruth Tucker was very ill and the surgeon asked her if she would risk a transplant.

'She was told that we couldn't promise her anything in the way of a cure,' he explains, 'and I made it clear that this procedure had never been performed successfully before. There was no push to try and make her do it, I'll tell you, none whatsoever. I wouldn't even take a direct answer. I told her: "You go home and think about it. Discuss it with your family."'[1]

Ruth Tucker agreed to give it a try. In May 1950, Richard

Lawler put the word out to other hospitals in Chicago and to the coroner's office that he was looking for a donor, a woman of much the same size and blood type as Ruth. He even approached the city's prison for a volunteer but gave up that idea when the warders insisted that his patient have her operation inside the jail to minimize the chance of an escape. 'We decided that it would be too tough on our patient, psychologically, to put her behind bars for the operation,' says Lawler. 'Then we waited. And, so help me, over the next six weeks very few emergency cases occurred that might have provided a usable kidney. For some reason, people must have been driving very carefully or behaving themselves during that period.'[2]

Ruth Tucker's anxieties grew as the weeks passed with no sign of a donor. She was desperate for the chance of life, but felt uneasy that her survival now depended on someone else's death. 'She would ask me to pray that there'd be a suitable kidney that someone would be able to give to her,' says Sister Joseph Casey, a student nurse in the hospital in 1950, who had been asked to look after Ruth before her operation. 'Her window was on the seventh floor overlooking the driveway into the emergency room. And when she heard an ambulance, she would turn to me and say: "I don't wish evil for anyone, but I certainly hope that maybe one of these days, there will be someone that could give me a kidney." '

Finally, in June, Lawler got word that the nearby Little Company of Mary Hospital had the donor he was looking for, a forty-nine-year-old woman in the last stages of cirrhosis of the liver. When she died, the patient's daughter gave Lawler permission to remove a kidney to save Ruth Tucker's life. On 17 June the two operations began simultaneously in adjacent operating theatres. The donor's kidney was removed and carried across the hall to the room where Richard Lawler had just excised Ruth's hugely swollen left kidney. The procedure took just forty-five minutes but, by the end, the room was packed with people who had come to see history made. 'We had up to forty doctors watching,' says Lawler. 'Some were even standing on tables in the back. A photographer that we hired to get a motion picture record of the procedure apparently was not accustomed to operations. Midway through he fainted dead away and one of the doctors in the audience had to take over the camera work.'[3]

As she lay in her hospital bed recovering from the anaesthetic, Ruth Tucker was the talk of the nation. The news pack descended on Chicago with a vengeance. 'Reporters gave me a hell of a lot of trouble,' Lawler explains, 'calling my home at any hour, day or night. Soon after the transplant it got so bad I moved into the hospital . . .'[4]

The enthusiasm of America's newspapers was understandable – although their apparent ignorance of Yu Yu Voronoy was less so. 'This is the first time . . . that a human organ has been transmitted from one person to another,'[5] proclaimed an editorial in the *New York Times*. According to *Time* magazine, the Chicago doctors had performed 'the first human kidney transplant on record'.[6] *Newsweek* added its voice to the inaccurate hyperbole. 'Up to last week,' wrote the magazine's medical correspondent, 'no vital human organ had ever been moved from one person to another.'[7]

But there was criticism too. Many thought Lawler had overstepped the mark. They wondered how he could justify operating on a patient after such poor results from his experimental animal transplants. They said the removal of the donor's kidney was a violation of a dead body. They complained that it wasn't sufficient simply to match the body size and blood type of the donor and recipient: tissue type had to be taken into account as well. One predicted that Lawler's patient would die of allergic shock. But Ruth Tucker didn't die. Her transplanted kidney began to function almost immediately. Against all the odds she got better, so much so that one month after her operation Tucker walked out of the hospital with her husband and went home to lead a normal life. It looked like a major triumph: for the first time rejection seemed beaten and a woman's life saved by a transplant.

Yet there was a snag. The doctors didn't know which of Ruth's kidneys was keeping her alive: was it the remaining diseased right kidney or the transplanted left one?

In April 1951, nearly ten months later, Lawler had the opportunity to find out. Ruth Tucker's kidneys were producing less and less urine, so he asked her to return to the Little Company of Mary Hospital for an exploratory operation. What Lawler found when he inspected the transplanted kidney was at odds with his patient's continued survival – but entirely in line with all that was then known about the biological force of rejection. 'It had diminished from normal size to about that of a large walnut. Although the tissues still looked alive, the organ was clearly not producing urine,' says Lawler.[8]

The kidney had been reduced to a small brownish-red lump and was no longer connected to the ureter, the tube that leads from the kidney to the bladder.[9] Rejection had once again exacted its toll, but Ruth Tucker lived on for another five years, dying in 1956 of a heart complaint. Exactly why she survived so long remains a mystery. Lawler thinks the transplant might have taken the load off her own kidney long enough to allow it to recover. Despite this, the American Urological Association held a press conference in 1951 to announce the failure of the transplant. 'Clinical evidence now shows,' it announced, 'that because of biological incompatibility of tissues, the kidney transplant operation cannot be advocated at present.'[10]

Although the gamble might have helped Ruth Tucker over a crisis, it had not been the breakthrough for which everyone had been hoping – and it did little for Lawler's career or his personal relationships in Chicago. 'I was ostracized by much of the profession,' he writes. 'There were so very few supporters. Some of my good friends wouldn't even talk to me for fear that I would contaminate them. I think some of this was due to the feeling at the time that doctors who got their names into the newspapers were trying to advertise themselves.'[11]

It was such a painful episode that Lawler never performed another transplant. To have done so, he says, would have been like waving a red rag to a bull. Yet his pioneering work had not been wasted: almost a year had passed before the failure of Ruth Tucker's transplant was revealed, and the ambiguity of her survival was a beacon of hope to other medical teams keen to pursue the transplant dream. Unwittingly, perhaps, Richard Lawler had fired the starting pistol of a transatlantic race between doctors in America and France to transplant the kidney. One of the front-runners was René Küss, a distinguished French surgeon then working at the Cochin Hospital in Paris. Küss is now eighty-three and one of the last survivors of the era.

'Lawler had an extraordinary impact on those of us in France who were doing experimental transplantation,' he says. 'It gave us the reason to believe that transplant surgery was possible in human beings . . . His results and his conclusions were not entirely convincing . . . but we were so anxious to apply the experience we had gathered working on dogs to human beings that we used Lawler's success as an excuse to begin kidney transplants in man.'

Two other teams of surgeons in France were in the running: one was led by Jean Hamburger, then the head of the nephrology department at the Necker Hospital in Paris, and the other by Charles Dubost and Marceau Servelle, two surgeons at the Broussais Hospital in Paris. The American effort was spearheaded by David Hume, another surgeon, at the Peter Bent Brigham Hospital in Boston.[12]

The atmosphere in France in 1951 was, if anything, even less conducive to transplantation than it was in America. The idea was dismissed outright on moral and practical grounds and French surgeons who wanted to make spare-part surgery a reality provoked just as much disapproval as Lawler had in America. 'Most people thought it was totally insane, just as they did after Carrel's experimentation,' says René Küss. 'They thought it was absolutely impossible to transcend the laws of nature by mixing two individuals, so public opinion was against this type of experimentation. They were convinced we were doomed to failure.'

Not surprisingly, the French found transplantable kidneys hard to come by. A few came from live donors, patients who were suffering from illnesses like hydrocephalus[13] or an inoperable narrowing of the ureter, who had been forced to have a healthy kidney removed. But such 'free' kidneys were rare, and moral disapproval ruled out the removal of organs from people who had died natural deaths.[14] Kidneys were in such short supply that transplantation might never have got off the ground in France – but for the discovery of a gruesome alternative supply. Surgeons in Paris received permission to take them from freshly executed prisoners. 'There was no choice. We had to go to the Santé Prison,' Charles Dubost says: 'I telephoned the director to ask whether or not they had an execution in the near future. He said, "Yes." I said, "Could I take his kidneys?" "Yes, sir. Without doubt. He'll be dead – without a head, so you can take the kidneys." '[15]

In January 1951, just over six months after Lawler's transplant, Dubost and Servelle took a trip down to the prison to await the execution of a prisoner. As soon as the guillotine had fallen, the two surgeons removed the organs from the unfortunate man's headless, bloody corpse and hurried back to the hospital. Dubost grafted one kidney into a forty-two-year-old woman. The new organ worked briefly but the patient died seventeen days later. Servelle put the other kidney into a twenty-two-year-old woman who fared no better, surviving for just nineteen days.

A week after that execution, René Küss did his first kidney transplant. He avoided the horrors of the Santé Prison, finding instead a healthy 'free' kidney.[16] But he had little more success than Dubost and Servelle: his patient died five weeks later.

The story of kidney transplantation in the first two years of the 1950s was one of failure and repeated failure. Küss tried four more times in 1951, but none of his transplants worked for more than a few weeks.[17] Jean Hamburger's team took their first step in 1952 when a sixteen-year-old carpenter arrived at the Necker Hospital with no kidneys: Marius Renard had fallen and damaged his right kidney so badly that it had to be removed. Soon afterwards, the boy discovered that he could not urinate. The reason, as his hapless surgeon soon discovered, was because Marius had been born with only one kidney which had now been excised. To save his life, his mother agreed to give one of her own kidneys to her son. It was transplanted on Christmas Day, the first voluntary live organ donation. The kidney was rejected twenty-one days later and Marius died a few days after that.[18]

The Americans began to transplant kidneys into patients in March 1951. The Peter Bent Brigham Hospital in Boston had a major advantage: they possessed one of the first artificial kidney machines. It wasn't sophisticated enough to keep patients alive indefinitely, but the Boston team thought it might improve their patients' condition before the transplant and give them a better chance of success.[19] It made little difference: David Hume transplanted kidneys into eight desperately ill people in 1951 and 1952,[20] which all failed. An atmosphere of gloom spread among the transplant teams.

'We learned that several other factors contributed to the failure of transplants,' says René Küss. 'For example, the weakened condition of the patient, inadequate intensive-care techniques and rampant infections all added to the biological rejection. We never really knew if it was simple rejection or if all these other complications were responsible for the failure. The results from medical teams in France as well as the United States led us to believe that transplant surgery was impossible.'

Hope was fast disappearing. Unlike Carrel, Jaboulay and Voronoy, this generation of surgeons and physicians had known their chances of success were not great. They understood the power of rejection and realized it would almost certainly doom transplants between genetically dissimilar individuals. Yet as patients were dying of incurable kidney diseases in their hospitals and as there were no other long-term means of helping them, it is hardly surprising they grasped at straws. They also knew that they could not continue indefinitely with such an experimental treatment without a real sign that it could work. They needed at least one victory to keep the dream alive. It came at the eleventh hour in Boston, and to this day no one knows the reason for the success.

Early in 1953, David Hume decided to transplant a kidney into his ninth patient, a twenty-six-year-old South American doctor who was suffering from Bright's disease.[21] The patient had first shown signs of the illness when he was twelve but was now in the last stages of kidney failure. His ankles were swollen, he suffered terrible headaches, he couldn't see properly, he vomited continually and his blood pressure had risen dangerously high. He didn't have long to live. In February 1953 a kidney removed from a patient who had died of heart failure was transplanted into the young man's right thigh, the position in which Hume chose to place nearly all his grafts during this period. Things went badly from the start.

'The patient showed a marked tendency to bleed abnormally,' writes Francis Moore, then surgeon-in-chief at the hospital. 'He required many blood transfusions. The transplant made no urine . . . Things looked very dark and the course did not seem much better than those of any of the previous patients.'

But nineteen days after the operation, the kidney began to work. The patient still had his own diseased kidneys, but because Hume had chosen to place the transplant in the patient's thigh, with its ureter poking out from a hole in the skin of his leg, it was possible to measure the organ's output. There was no ambiguity this time: it was the transplanted kidney that was keeping him alive. At last, half a century after the first attempt to transplant a kidney, there appeared to be a chink in the impenetrable armour of rejection.

'The patient got out of bed and began to walk around. His appetite returned and he gained weight . . . He was discharged on the eighty-first day after transplantation, the first patient in history to be discharged from hospital living solely on the function of a kidney taken from another person,' says Moore.

Eventually, the patient's health worsened again: he developed a fever, his leg began to swell and the transplanted kidney slowly failed. He died on 8 June 1953, five days short of six months after his operation. But, thanks to Hume's transplanted kidney, he had been given the precious gift of 176 days of renewed life and vigour. 'It was incredible,' continues Moore. 'Almost six months . . . And when he got his disease again and knew he was going to die he said: "I hope my experience will help others as much as it has helped me." He was very grateful for his six months of life. And he died.'

The transplanted kidney had been destroyed by the high blood pressure that was a feature of his illness and which the doctors had been unable to lower. When Hume looked at the kidney after the man's death he discovered little evidence of rejection.[22] It is now thought that the reason for this was a rare and lucky match between the tissue type of the donor and that of the recipient, but at the time, the reason for his patient's long survival was a mystery to Hume, which perhaps explains the gloomy assessment of his nine transplants. 'At the present state of our knowledge,' he wrote, 'renal homotransplants[23] do not appear to be justified in the treatment of human disease.'[24]

It was an understandable prognosis in an experimental field that had suffered so many failures, but Hume's one partial success breathed new life into a treatment that many believed was destined to fail. If one person could be kept alive for six months on a transplanted kidney, it was reasonable to suppose that others could as well.

'Doctors who take care of patients have to be optimists and will seize any possible glimmer of hope to help patients,' explains Joseph Murray, who continued the transplant work at Boston when Hume left the hospital in 1953.[25] 'Because kidney disease often affected young people and the kidneys were the only diseased organs in these patients, it was tempting to replace them. Somehow, intuitively, you felt that if we could only do this, it would work. So this human experience was very conducive to keeping the optimism going. We felt that physiologically and mechanically we could succeed.'

A lucky break, though, however laudable, was not sufficient. If twenty or thirty grafts had to fail before one patient was allowed a few months of renewed life, the stakes were still far too high. Success had to be predictable and survival times measured in years if transplantation were to progress from a high-risk experiment to a life-saving treatment. For the moment, the initiative in the race to transplant the kidney stayed with the American team in Boston where Joseph Murray found a way of ensuring the success and predictability he so desired. But there was a price to pay. Kidney transplants could be made to work but only by limiting them to an exceptionally small and exclusive group of people: identical twins, those resulting from a single fertilized egg that has split into two in the womb.

In 1954 Dr David C. Miller of the United States Public Health Service telephoned the transplant team at the Peter Bent Brigham Hospital to tell them that he had a patient, Richard Herrick, suffering from chronic kidney failure. This wasn't an unusual occurrence: word of the hospital's transplant programme had spread far and wide and, despite the attrition rate, the team was inundated with sick people clamouring for treatment. But this call was different, for Dr Miller knew a little about transplantation. He knew, for example, that rejection should not be a problem between genetically identical individuals because a transplanted organ would not be seen as 'foreign' by the recipient's body. Richard Herrick, he told the hospital, had a brother, Ronald, who was his identical twin.

'I couldn't believe it,' Murray recollects. 'We were just beside ourselves. We couldn't believe we were going to have a chance to do a transplant with no immunological barrier.'

Richard Herrick had been five years old when he caught scarlet fever. The disease is rarely serious nowadays, thanks to the use of penicillin, but before the use of antibiotics, it could damage the kidneys. Richard got over his illness and was quite healthy until he was twenty-two, when his legs and feet began to swell. Tests showed that his blood pressure was high as was the level of waste products in his blood, both classic signs of kidney failure. He was suffering from Bright's disease and by the time he was admitted to the Peter Bent Brigham Hospital in 1954 he had no chance of survival.

Murray was convinced he could save Richard's life with one of Ronald's kidneys. If he got the surgery right, there should be no rejection and therefore no reason for it to fail – and he would prove beyond doubt the feasibility of transplantation. But to do so, Murray and his surgical colleagues had to step into a moral minefield. They would be operating on someone who did not need an operation. The removal of Ronald's healthy kidney might save his brother's life but it couldn't possibly benefit Ronald. In effect, the team would risk the health of one patient for the sake of someone else. It was an acute dilemma. One of the most fundamental principles of the medical profession can be expressed very simply: 'Do no harm.' All doctors accept this precept and carry it with them throughout their professional lives. Jean Hamburger's transplant team had faced the same issue in Paris in 1952 when they had tried to save young Marius Renard's life with a graft from his mother. Now, in 1954, the chance to save life with an organ donated by a living person once again seemed to threaten this most sacrosanct of maxims.

'It was against all the dicta of being a physician: to do no harm,' says Murray. 'We were doing a lot of harm and we all felt very strongly about it. We were concerned. We discussed it with clergy of all faiths. We consulted physicians in other hospitals. We had lawyers come in. We had members of the general public. We talked to an awful lot of people. One of them said: "If it's reasonable to lay down your life for your fellow man it is certainly reasonable to give an organ." That person had a very global view which transcended our medical view.'

But there was opposition too. Some physicians felt that such an operation was wrong in principle and that, anyway, it probably wouldn't work. One of Murray's close friends at the hospital, another surgeon, told him bluntly that the planned transplant would ruin his career. The arguments were rehearsed and re-rehearsed, and Murray withstood several sleepless nights before making up his mind to go ahead. The decision was even more difficult for Ronald Herrick, who was being asked to sacrifice one of his kidneys. 'I was a little bit taken aback by the thought because . . . it had never been done before and when you're the one who might be doing it, why it takes you aback, I can tell you that,' he explains. 'It isn't something that you want to take lightly. Because here I was, I felt fine and while I wanted to help my brother, I suppose you think of yourself first . . . I wasn't impressed with the idea, particularly at first.'

Murray told Ronald that he could live a long and healthy life with just one kidney. But Ronald needed reassurance. The turning point came during a meeting between the transplant team and the twins. 'I'll never forget it,' he says. 'There were about five of us, key physicians, in the room with the family. The donor asked: 'If I go through with this, will you, the hospital, be responsible for my health for the rest of my life?' Dr Harrison, the surgeon who would be operating on the donor and who therefore bore the most responsibility, said: 'Ronald, of course not. But do you think that anybody in this room would refuse to take care of you if you came in?' It was very telling because Ronald realized that his future didn't rest in some legalism but in the integrity of the profession. It was a decisive moment.'

Before performing the operation, Murray had to be sure that Richard was Ronald's identical twin. They looked identical – they even had the same birthmark on one of their ears – but one was a little taller than the other. Murray swapped skin grafts between the two men: only if they were truly identical twins would the grafts survive. They did. He also found out that their fingerprint patterns were identical. 'I didn't know how to take fingerprints,' he remembers, 'so I called up the police and they said: "Sure, we'll be glad to fingerprint the patients. What do you want this for?" Now I didn't realize there were police reporters around so I mentioned that we were thinking of transplanting a kidney from one twin to the other. That day, going home from the hospital, I turned on the car radio and I got the news that Brigham doctors were planning a daring operation! The cat was out of the bag.' A media jamboree descended on the Peter Bent Brigham Hospital with reporters who were every bit as dogged in their pursuit of the story as they had been in Chicago four years earlier. 'We'd even find out on the radio, on our way in to work in the mornings, what the blood count of our patient was because the media had paid off some of the night staff at the hospital. They found out everything from them,' says Murray.

Much was resting on the success of the Herrick transplant: after the string of failures in both America and France, transplantation would suffer a terrible blow if Joseph Murray was unable to keep Richard alive with Ronald's kidney. Murray was well aware of the significance of what he was about to attempt. He had already carried out several unsuccessful human kidney transplants between genetically dissimilar individuals,[26] and while he had done scores of transplants in dogs, he had never put the kidney behind the appendix. He wanted to place Richard's new organ here because it was a relatively easy part of the body to reach and in which to join the blood vessels together. Since he was suffering from first-night nerves and had to be certain he would get it right, Murray went down to the hospital mortuary and practised the new technique on a body awaiting autopsy.

The transplant was planned for 24 December 1954. On the night before, Richard's conscience began to plague him. Was it fair, he wondered, for his brother to sacrifice a kidney for him? Was this asking too much of fraternal love? Ronald was already in the hospital when Richard rang him to say that he did not want to have the transplant, that he would rather die. But Ronald's mind was made up. 'I said, well, I'm already here so we're going to do it – and that's it. I think he felt there was too much risk involved for me, but I didn't feel that way at that point. I felt it was the best thing to do for the both of us.'

On Christmas Eve, the world's first identical-twin kidney transplant took place at the Peter Bent Brigham Hospital in Boston. It was a crucial moment in the history of transplant surgery. A success would not solve the problem of rejection – but it would be a step towards realizing the dream of spare part surgery. 'If the operation had failed,' says Murray, 'transplantation as a discipline would have been set back years, maybe decades, because there was an inherent feeling against the whole concept.'

But Ronald's generous gift survived – and took an immediate liking to its new home inside his brother's body. 'The transplanted kidney was making nice, clean, clear, yellow urine,' explains Francis Moore. 'Although you may never have developed any affection for urine, if you or your parents are unable to make any, you come to appreciate it.'[27]

Its effect on Richard Herrick was dramatic. 'Before the operation, his heart had been enlarged and there was fluid in his lungs,' Moore continues. 'Within a few weeks the heart had decreased in size, the fluid in the lungs cleared and clinical progress was good with return of appetite, strength and vigour. Within a month the patient was on the road to convalescence.'[28]

Ronald – who suffered no ill effects from the removal of his kidney – was astonished at the sudden restoration of good health in his brother. 'It was remarkable how his gaunt, yellow look changed to him looking like a normal person,' he says. 'It was only a few days and he looked much, much better . . . It was just beyond description, really. Here was a person who wasn't going to make it, who appeared to be making it. Everyone in the family was happy.'

Several weeks after the transplant Richard's own diseased kidneys were removed to help bring his blood pressure down to normal. Then he went home, married the nurse who had looked after him during his stay in hospital and took up his work again as a radio and TV engineer. Richard had eight years of good health that he could not possibly have expected without the transplant. He died in 1963 of coronary artery disease, after a recurrence of the Bright's disease in his new kidney. Today Ronald continues to live a normal life on his one remaining kidney. The gamble had paid off: the gift had given life without harming the donor. It was proof positive that transplant surgery could be a life-saver. Yet ultimately the victory was only a technical one: the Boston transplant team had demonstrated that, with the correct surgical procedure, transplantation could succeed, as long as rejection was not a problem. But a therapy limited to identical twins was regarded by many doctors as little more than a medical curiosity. Rejection had to be tackled, not bypassed, if spare-part surgery was ever to become a mainstream medical treatment. Despite the world-wide publicity it attracted, the Herrick transplant provided no answers to the main obstacle on the path to progress.

Perhaps fate decrees that great discoveries occur only when sufficient people are willing them to happen, the desires of many combining to provide the right intellectual backdrop for the breakthrough. Or maybe it is only coincidence. Whatever the reason, the first scientific advance in the battle against rejection took place at precisely the time that it was most needed. While surgeons in America and France were trying to bludgeon the immune system into submission by transplanting kidneys and hoping for the best, the British scientist Peter Medawar hit upon a more subtle and effective approach: trickery. The idea came to him after he visited a herd of cows on an experimental farm near Birmingham. A colleague had asked him to help to find a way of distinguishing between cattle that were identical twins and those that were fraternal twins, resulting from two separate fertilized eggs and which are not therefore genetically identical. Medawar knew that skin could only be transplanted successfully between two individuals if they were genetically identical so he suggested exchanging such grafts between the twin calves. If they were rejected, then the animals must be fraternal; if they were accepted, the twins would be identical. It seemed an elegant and simple solution. There was one problem. It didn't work.

'The results were not at all what we had expected,' writes Medawar, 'since *all* cattle twins accepted skin grafts one from another for as long as we had them under observation. Some of these twins must certainly have been non-identical because they were of different sexes. These results were totally anomalous . . .'[29]

Why should skin transplanted between non-identical cattle twins be spared the ravages of rejection when the text-books said it should be quickly destroyed? In solving this mystery, Medawar laid the second foundation stone of his new science of immunology and, at the same time, discovered the first reliable method of preventing the immune system from attacking transplanted tissue. It was the breakthrough that everyone had been wanting – yet paradoxically it appeared of little practical help to the surgeons who most needed it.

While they are in the womb, the blood of one fraternally twinned calf mixes with that of the other because the two embryos have a shared placenta.[30] Medawar realized that this mixing of blood must happen before the immune system has developed, before it can recognize the other twin's blood as 'foreign'. By sneaking in early, so to speak, the blood cells were not rejected when the immune system matured. But if blood cells from the fraternal twin were now treated as if they were the animal's own cells, the immune system should be unable to distinguish any of the tissues of one twin from the other. This,

Medawar reasoned, was why the skin grafts survived and if rejection can be beaten by an accident of nature, he thought that it should not be beyond the wit of man to do the same in the laboratory. 'Our ambition was to bring about by design the immunological phenomenon that occurs naturally in twin cattle, namely to reduce, even abolish, their power to recognize and destroy genetically foreign tissues,' he writes.[31]

Working with two colleagues, Leslie Brent and Rupert Billingham, in the zoology department of University College in London, he experimented to see if he could prevent brown mice from rejecting skin transplanted onto their backs from a different strain of white mouse. He injected cells from the white mouse into baby brown mice, either just before or immediately after they were born. 'We'd worked quite hard for the best part of a year before we had the first glimpse that tolerance could be induced in mice,' recalls Leslie Brent. 'It was extraordinarily exciting when we realized that the skin was not being rejected.'

Medawar and his co-workers eventually had brown mice running around their laboratory bearing skin grafts from white mice. They did the same successfully with chickens. A big hole had been punched in the force that so unremittingly destroyed organ grafts between genetically dissimilar individuals. They had shown that rejection could be halted and their supermice caused a sensation at a time when many scientists thought that such a biological solution to rejection was not possible. But was this just an interesting laboratory observation or could it help surgeons in the struggle to save those otherwise doomed by chronic kidney failure? It was one thing to inject foreign tissues into unborn mice, quite another to contemplate doing the same in unborn human children. It was neither practically nor morally acceptable: memories of the Nazis' abhorrent wartime medical experiments were still uncomfortably fresh in people's minds. It was also clear that the technique could not help patients now dying of kidney disease. Sir Roy Calne, the English transplant surgeon, remembers Medawar's frank approach to this issue. 'Medawar was a most brilliant speaker,' he says, 'and he came in with his perfectly delivered lecture and showed the most fantastic pictures of brown mice with white skin grafts and black chickens with white feathers. At the end of this wonderful lecture, one of the students asked him if he felt there would be any application of his work in the treatment of patients. He paused for a moment and then smiled and answered with two words: "Absolutely none".'

But this was only half the truth. Medawar's discovery galvanized the transplant community. At a time when despair was dominant, it gave surgeons and researchers renewed hope that a practical solution to rejection could be found. Looking back on this period with the benefit of hindsight, Medawar fully appreciated the impact of his work. 'The ultimate importance of the discovery of tolerance turned out to be not practical but moral,' he wrote in 1986. 'It put new heart into the many biologists and surgeons who were working to make it possible to graft, for example, kidneys from one person to another . . .'[32]

Medawar's patchwork mice and Murray's success with identical twins gave the transplant teams in America and France the theoretical and surgical justification they needed to try again to tackle rejection. They realized that it was no good just to transplant a kidney and hope for the best, that they had to find some means of weakening the biological force of rejection. The method most opted for was 'total body irradiation'. Studies of the victims of the atomic bombs dropped on Hiroshima and Nagasaki had shown that survivors seemed much more suscept- ible to illness. X-ray radiation appeared to weaken the body's immune system, preventing it from attacking and killing foreign invaders. But if X-rays can lower resistance to bacteria and viruses, the transplanters thought they might have the same effect against the immune system's ability to destroy a transplanted organ. In theory, it seemed sound. In practice, it was like using a sledgehammer to crack a nut.

American surgeons began to test X-rays on transplanted rabbits, dogs and mice. There were usually three steps to the procedure: first, the animals were given enough X-rays to destroy all the cells in the lymph nodes, the bone marrow and the spleen which normally attack a transplant. Then they were injected with fresh bone-marrow cells taken from other donors to provide a new immune system that, they believed, would not attack the future graft. Finally they received the transplant. Francis Moore calls this the 'beachhead' concept of grafting: 'bombardment first with irradiation, then a shore party of bone-marrow cells to prepare the way for the main invasion by kidney' is his graphic description of the procedure.[33]

Hundreds of animal experiments in Boston resulted in a handful of survivors, their additional life-span measured in weeks rather than years. It was hardly the most promising basis on which to restart clinical work. But Murray, Hamburger and Küss faced the same dilemma that had provoked the first series of kidney transplants: the presence of terminally ill patients in their hospitals for whom there was no other form of treatment. Another series of human kidney transplants began: at the Peter Bent Brigham Hospital in 1958, and a few months later in Paris, using X-rays to try to control rejection.

The first person to undergo the treatment was Gladys Lowman, an American who arrived in Boston with no kidneys. Her brother, Roy Dalton, remembers how she came to be in this dire predicament. 'I went to visit sis and she said, "Roy, feel this knot on my side here." And that was the first time that I knew she was sick. The next day she was rushed to the hospital and they . . . found out it was her kidney and they didn't have any choice but to take it out because it was in such bad shape. Well, they kept waiting for her [other] kidney to work and it didn't. So they checked and that's how they found out she didn't have any.'

The surgeon who had removed Gladys Lowman's diseased kidney had not realized that she was one of the few people born each year with only one kidney. She was now under sentence of death: even with the help of the early artificial kidney machine she would be unable to survive for more than a week or two. A transplant was her only hope and Joseph Murray decided to see if X-rays would prevent her body from destroying the new organ. 'We explained to her and to her family the protocol of using total body X-ray and bone-marrow replacement,' says Murray. 'She . . . was delighted that there was at least a possibility. And that was a common theme we had from the patients referred during those years. The only other alternative was to give up and die. And many patients would say: "I'm happy to try it, even though it's an experiment and it may not help me but it will help others in the future." That was a universal comment.'

Lowman was placed on her side underneath an X-ray machine and given a high enough dose of irradiation[34] to destroy all her bone marrow, which was then replaced with bone marrow taken from her five brothers and six other donors who had flown into Boston to help save her life. It was a vital part of the procedure – but exceptionally painful. The marrow was removed with a large needle pushed into the donors' hips. A local anaesthetic was used to dull the pain, but Gladys Lowman's brothers still cannot recall the event without wincing. '[It was the] most painful thing I ever had done to me in my life,' Roy Dalton recalls. 'It's a fact that if I live for ever, I won't be hurt that bad. I went through other serious things but nothing like this pain. . . . Your knees would pop and, oh, you'd scream. In fact, they thought I'd passed out on them and they went over and raised my eyelid to see if I was still with them.'

Another brother, Fred, also remembers the agony. 'They drilled holes inside three places in your femur bone,' he says, 'and the next day you couldn't get up. Someone had to help you get out of the chair. Scabs as big as your thumb would heal over where they'd done this. I mean it's really crude, really crude.'

After the transplant, Lowman lay in her carefully sterilized hospital room praying for a miracle. The artificial kidney was removing just enough waste from her blood to keep her alive but if the transplant was rejected, she would be overwhelmed. For two weeks, the new organ stubbornly refused to do its job. Then, suddenly, it began to remove the poisons building up in her body. Murray and the transplant team breathed a sigh of relief – but they quickly discovered there was no cause for celebration. Her donors' bone marrow didn't take and Gladys Lowman was left defenceless against the most minor infections. Twenty-eight days after her operation she died.

'We were very enthused for the first month because we thought this was going to be it . . . [But] she succumbed to infection and bleeding,' says Joseph Murray. 'The side-effects resulting from the lack of marrow, were lethal . . . But looking at the kidney microscopically, it was functioning and no sign of rejection.'

Two things became clear over the next three years: first, X-rays did the trick – with sufficient irradiation, transplanted kidneys showed few signs of rejection; second, most of the patients died soon after their operations because irradiation so weakened their immune systems that they were left wide open to infections the body normally shrugs off. In short, the kidney lived but the patients died, killed by something as simple as the common cold before they could benefit from their transplant.

Joseph Murray grafted kidneys into ten people after treating them with total body irradiation.[35] Nine died within a month of their operations. René Küss did three transplants using the technique to stop rejection; two died within days of their transplants[36] and the third lived for four and a half months. Four of Jean Hamburger's six irradiation patients lived a similarly short time. Amid the failures, however, there were a few spectacular successes. One of Murray's patients, John Riteris, lived for twenty years with his non-identical twin brother's kidney inside him. One of Hamburger's, a postman called Georges Siméon, lived for twenty-five years after receiving a new organ from his non-identical twin brother.[37] X-rays, then, had given surgeons a means of breaking the genetic barrier but only between exceptionally closely related individuals and then only rarely. The successes were notable precisely because they were the exceptions. The rule was still failure and early death.

'This was a terribly bad period for us,' Francis Moore recalls. 'Our high-dose X-ray experiences were pretty disastrous . . . We were sent patients from all over the world, often with no kidneys and we operated on them. But they failed. And that's what I call the black period.'

Transplantation had reached another impasse. Surgeons using X-rays walked a razor-sharp knife-edge: too much irradiation and the patient was overwhelmed by infection; too little and the transplant was destroyed by rejection. There was no margin for error. Joseph Murray kept a depressing tally. 'At least eighteen

normal kidneys have been removed from healthy volunteer
donors to achieve an aggregate of forty-five extra months of life
for five individuals,' he wrote in 1962. 'This balance sheet should
caution everyone contemplating further use of this approach in
human transplantation.'[38]

That is where the transplant story might have ended but for the
efforts of Roy (now Sir Roy) Calne, the English surgeon who
wouldn't take no for an answer. The slow death of a young
patient in Guy's Hospital in 1951[39] had sparked off his lifelong
interest in the idea of swapping of new organs for old. Calne
followed the developments in transplant surgery with growing
interest while serving with the British Army's Royal Medical
Corps in Hong Kong and Malaysia. When he returned to civilian
life in the mid 1950s, he began his own experiments on dogs at
the Royal Free Hospital in London. It was clear that without a safe
and reliable method of preventing rejection, public opinion
would soon turn against transplantation. 'The urgent need for
kidney transplantation,' he wrote of this period in 1964, 'is a
source of concern to clinicians and of distress to patients and
their relatives, especially in view of the immense publicity that
some attempts at clinical transplantation have received.'[40]

Time was short. Calne's experiments convinced him that
X-rays were a dead-end approach, and he wondered whether
drugs being used to prevent cancer might provide a better means
of suppressing the immune system and hence controlling
rejection. A colleague told him about a promising anti-leukaemia
drug 6-mercaptopurine (6-MP).[41] Laboratory tests had already
shown[42] that 6-MP could weaken the immune system in rabbits,
and Calne thought it might do the same in his transplanted dogs.
He obtained a supply, tested it in London, and soon had dogs
living up to five times as long as before.[43] But he quickly
discovered that England was not the best place for experimental
research. 'Trying to do research in a surgical subject in 1959 in
London was even more difficult than it is now,' he says. 'There
were no resources. There was no encouragement. Most people
tended to regard anybody who wanted to do this kind of thing as
rather crazy. My boss at the Royal Free Hospital . . . warned the

ward sister that she needed to watch that I didn't put animals in the beds because I seemed to be doing a lot of experimental work. This was the attitude in England at that time.'

Calne decided to take his own supply of the new drug to America,[44] joining Joseph Murray's team in Boston shortly after they began their own experiments with 6-MP. He spent most of 1960 working in the animal laboratories at the Peter Bent Brigham Hospital. Operating on his dogs, caring for them and testing the function of their transplanted kidneys was a full-time occupation that required a dedication beyond the call of duty. 'I used to collect urine from the dogs,' he says. 'It's not very difficult to collect urine from a male dog but the speed and co-ordination needed to collect urine from a female is very exacting and you need to train for it! The bitch doesn't give any notice that she's about to pass urine and my friends and colleagues used to call it the 'Calne Crouch', the way you'd have to suddenly crouch under the dog to collect the urine.'

It was undignified but Calne's commitment paid off. He demonstrated that 6-MP and a closely related chemical called Imuran[45] were a safer means of preventing rejection in his animals than irradiation. The star of his laboratory was a dog called Lollipop, presented in 1960 to an academic audience in the auditorium at the Peter Bent Brigham Hospital alive and well six months after a kidney transplant and treatment with Imuran. 'Lollipop was delighted to be let loose in this environment,' he recalls, 'and licked all the important professors in the front row of the huge auditorium there. I'm sure they won't forget it.'

It was time to go back to the clinic. The third major attempt since 1951 to force the body to accept the gift of life began in Boston in April 1960 and in Paris two months after that. Murray, Küss and Hamburger tried the new drug therapy on increasing numbers of transplant patients. The French combined the chemicals with X-rays; the Americans used only the drugs. The verdict was clear: 6-MP and Imuran provided a far better means of controlling rejection. Where X-rays alone could offer only a knife-edge of survival, the drugs gave doctors a narrow ledge on which to walk. It became possible to halt rejection without exposing patients to overwhelming infection. Now transplant surgery had a realistic chance of becoming a regular therapy for irreversible kidney failure.

As surgeons began to break out of the genetic strait-jacket that the immune system had imposed upon them, the possibilities began to expand. No longer was transplantation limited to people with twin brothers or sisters. The new drugs enabled surgeons to keep some patients alive with kidneys taken from unrelated dead bodies.

René Küss was the first to save a patient's life in this way. In June 1960 he transplanted a twenty-six-year-old dying woman with a kidney donated by her brother-in-law. He used a combination of 6-MP and X-rays to prolong her life for seventeen months. In December 1961 he gave a second desperately ill patient eighteen months of useful life[46] with a kidney from a stranger. Joseph Murray's team in Boston claimed the third success in April 1962 when they kept a terminally ill young accountant alive for twenty-one months with a kidney taken from a man who had died during open heart surgery.[47]

The new drug therapy extended the lives of these patients by keeping their immune systems muzzled, while allowing them just enough rope to fight off infection. It was a delicate balancing act. The natural process of rejection was curtailed but, in most patients, not stopped. A slow but unremitting war of attrition continued inside their bodies until eventually the immune system would win: the kidney failed and the victim died.

Press coverage focused mainly on the successes and, as word of the new medical science spread across the globe, more and more desperate patients asked about transplants. It was in this febrile atmosphere that the pioneers decided it was time to compare notes. In September 1963, a select group of about twenty-five doctors and researchers from America, France, Britain and Canada met at the National Research Council building in Washington DC for a progress report. The results were not encouraging. The press and the public were clamouring for success but the doctors could offer only qualifications and inconsistency. Yes, they could do it now, they could keep patients alive with a transplant. Drugs could prevent rejection and had produced some stunning successes. But far too many patients still died early deaths to permit kidney grafts to become a regular treatment. A survey taken during this period[48] showed that, on average, less than 10 per cent of transplant patients lived as long as three months after their operations. Speaker after speaker demonstrated that success was like the ephemeral will-o'-the-wisp: so near yet always just out of reach.

And then Tom Starzl, the new boy at the meeting, took the stand. He had only begun doing kidney transplants in November 1962 at the Veterans' Administration Hospital in Denver, Colorado, and had not even been on the meeting's original invitation list. His attendance was an afterthought but he remembers the scene well. 'I found it difficult to speak. It may have been my insecurity in the presence of such important dignitaries which caused me to be uneasy. In addition, I felt like someone who had parachuted unannounced from another planet onto turf that was already occupied.'[49] Starzl had performed thirty-three kidney transplants. When he found his tongue, his results were met with disbelief. He had thought that this might be the case and, to convince the doubters, had brought with him the wall charts of his patients. Where the pioneers in the field were reporting uniformly high failure rates, twenty-seven of Starzl's patients were still alive with functioning kidneys at the time of the meeting.[50] 'I realized that we had more surviving kidney-transplant recipients by far than everyone else in the world combined,' he writes.[51]

Sir Roy Calne was at the meeting and well remembers the astonishment that greeted Starzl's results. 'I remember going through every case from Denver in a hotel room with Dr Starzl,' he says. 'He was an obsessional smoker at the time and I recall a pyramid of cigarette butts nearly two feet high. In between smoking he showed those flow-charts and they were so well worked out. It was the first time I had seen the systematic day-to-day assessment of results . . . and I think that was an extremely important contribution in terms of making the results overall better.'

Starzl had achieved his results by using a combination of drugs to keep rejection at bay. In common with all the other transplant teams, he had used Imuran to ward off rejection, but whenever their bodies showed signs of mounting an attack against the graft, he also gave his patients high doses of a steroid called Prednisone. The combination of these drugs proved much more powerful than when they were used individually.[52] Starzl described Prednisone's effect as 'almost miraculous'. 'Temperature returns to normal within a few hours and there is usually prompt evidence of improved renal function,'[53] he says.

It was now obvious that a carefully worked out cocktail of drugs could significantly subdue the onslaught of rejection. As doctors became more experienced at judging the doses, survival times grew longer. In a few of these early unrelated kidney transplants, it seemed as if drugs could win a permanent victory over rejection, but there was frequently a very high price to pay.

Yvette Thibault is one of the longest surviving transplant patients in the world. She was thirty-one in 1964 when she received a kidney from an unrelated donor. At the time she was dying of Bright's disease from which she had been suffering since she was a teenager. 'I was continually bleeding,' she recalls, from her second-floor flat in Paris. 'I couldn't get up. I couldn't go shopping. I was in a pitiful state . . . I was in such horrible pain I can't even describe it. I remember once going to a church to pray for some relief from the pain. Sometimes it would stop for a quarter of an hour. For me, a quarter of an hour of relief was like being in heaven.'

Yvette's life had been dogged by the illness: her body would swell; she could eat only certain foods; she became unbearably tired; she was forever having to go to the lavatory and her frequent stays in hospital meant she could never hold down a job for long. She is a courageous woman who did her best to live a normal life. When she became pregnant and was advised to have an abortion on the grounds that childbirth was likely to kill her, she had the baby anyway and survived. When she fell desperately ill on holiday in Brittany with her young son and had to return to the Necker Hospital in Paris, she refused to take an ambulance.

She was so sick she could hardly move but she didn't want to waste her return rail ticket.

'We knew her well,' says Jean Hamburger, who attended Yvette when she arrived at the hospital, 'because she had been hospitalized more than twelve times during the previous twelve years. We had been helpless witnesses to the progressive aggravation of her renal insufficiency. She was now practically unconscious, vomiting [and] almost blind . . .'[54]

Hamburger's surgical team transplanted Yvette in October 1964 and some weeks later her own diseased kidneys were removed. Her recovery was slow with many complications, but Yvette's stubborn will to live brought her safely through endless crises. Eventually, the transplanted kidney turned a living death into a new life. Since then Yvette has been – and still is – entirely dependent on the graft and the drugs[55] she receives each day to prevent rejection. Every time her immune system launches an attack on the kidney, Yvette's therapy is adjusted to deal with the problem. At one point she was taking fifty pills a day.

However, the power of the drugs keeping her alive is a double-edged sword: Yvette owes her life to them but the steroids have distorted her features. 'I started growing a beard and a moustache and at the same time I was becoming bald,' she explains. 'That was a traumatic experience because when you are out in the street it's absolutely awful – everyone laughs at you, you feel like a monster. It's really devastating.'

The drug dosage was reduced to minimize these side-effects but, in the long term, the physical effects of steroids, Imuran and other chemicals have been debilitating. Yvette has had skin cancer that has required extensive skin grafting. Severe pain in her knee joints forced her to spend a year in a wheelchair. She has also had triple by-pass surgery on her heart to cure arteriosclerosis, a disease that is also thought to have been provoked by her drug therapy. Yvette is frail and walks with a slight stoop but she passes off these problems as minor inconveniences. She is more than grateful for the thirty-two years of borrowed time that her transplanted kidney has given her. 'I often think about the person who gave me his kidney,' she says. 'I know that his initials were R.G. and that he was forty-two years old. I don't know what he died of but . . . his generosity has allowed me to live and that's very important. For me my birthdate doesn't count. My real birthday is 17 October 1964. That's when I started living a normal life – even if there were complications, even if I still have problems. I'll always feel that way, until the very end.'

By the mid 1960s, the slow, painful birth of kidney transplantation was almost completed. Thanks to the persistence of a handful of pioneers in America, France and Britain, spare-part surgery had become a reality after little more than a decade of concentrated effort. The hole that radiation had punched in the once impenetrable barrier of rejection had, with chemical immuno-suppression, become a yawning gulf. Lives were now being saved by a technique previously dismissed as fantasy. By any standards it was a great medical triumph and it is hardly surprising that, thirty years later, the Nobel committee in Stockholm decided to break with protocol and award its 1990 prize for medicine to a transplant surgeon. The accolade is usually reserved for those who have made great theoretical discoveries, but the enormous life-saving benefits of transplantation persuaded the committee to honour the practical skills of Joseph Murray.[56] They announced the decision in Stockholm at 11 a.m. on 8 October 1990.

It was 4 a.m. in San Francisco, where Murray was visiting his daughter. 'She woke me up,' says Murray, 'and said: "Daddy. I'm sorry to wake you but I have good news. You've won the Nobel Prize." I thought I was dreaming.'[57]

When the French read the news, they thought they were dreaming too. It wasn't that they believed Joseph Murray was an unworthy recipient of such a great honour but they wondered why the Nobel committee had so conspicuously ignored their own extensive contribution to the field of transplant surgery. The British had been honoured in 1960 when Peter Medawar received his Nobel Prize. Now they had honoured the Americans for work that 'paved the way for transplantation in man'.[58] 'We can't help but be surprised by the decision of the Nobel jury,' complained an editorial in *Le Monde* in 1990, 'because in 1952 the team working under the direction of Professor Jean Hamburger at the Necker Hospital was the first to achieve a prolonged survival of a kidney transplant from mother to son. It wasn't until 1954 that . . . Murray . . . managed to transplant a kidney between identical twins.'[59]

One of Hamburger's colleagues at the Necker Hospital was even more outspoken when asked for his reaction by a medical journalist. 'While we can be proud that Professor Murray was awarded the Nobel Prize,' he told *Le Quotidien du Médicine*, 'we deplore the fact that Professor Hamburger was not associated with this nomination.'[60]

Joseph Murray's Nobel Lecture,[61] delivered two months after receiving his award, succeeded only in rubbing salt into an open wound. He gave a short history of the first successful transplants and claimed a 'world's first' for the patient he had kept alive for twenty-one months from April 1962 with an unrelated-kidney transplant. There was no mention of René Küss's seventeen- and eighteen-month successes in June 1960 and December 1961.[62] Neither did Yvette Thibault's name pass his lips. Jean Hamburger couldn't contain his anger. As he wrote in a letter to a colleague shortly after the announcement of Murray's prize:

> I hate discussing priorities in scientific discoveries. But I cannot hide my surprise when I see some papers suggesting that renal transplantation was first successful in the United States. The group in Boston was first with identical twins, but this only requires a good surgical technique, and my group achieved kidney transplantation with excellent surgical results long before Murray and the Boston group . . . Of course I refused to answer the many journalists asking me to comment about Joe Murray's Nobel Prize since I like Joe very much. But frankly, between you and me, we did not understand in France the choice of the jury.[63]

No one had had the heart to tell Hamburger[64] that one reason why the Nobel committee had excluded the French was the bad feeling that existed between the two main transplant teams in Paris: Jean Hamburger and René Küss did not get on with each other and the committee knew that they would be stirring up trouble if they favoured one over the other. They chose the easy option, leaving France out of the reckoning altogether and generating considerable bad feeling themselves as a result.

'Nobel Prizes are a very difficult area and Nobel committees make mistakes and errors of commission and omission,' says Leslie Brent, the English immunologist, who wrote to Jean Hamburger expressing his regrets after the announcement of the prize. 'I didn't think that particular prize was put together terribly well. I would have been happier if the French contribution to the early pioneering days of kidney transplantation had been recognized by the Nobel Committee so I think I would have been happier to have seen Murray and Hamburger, who was still alive at that time, and Küss to have been joint Nobel Laureates for their role in kidney transplantation.'

With kidney transplantation now set to become the life-saver that everyone wanted it to be, surgeons naturally turned their attentions to other organs. If it can be done with the kidney, they reasoned, then why not with the liver or the heart? Francis Moore in Boston and Tom Starzl in Denver began to search for a way of saving lives with a transplanted liver. This effort was just as difficult and painstaking as had been the struggle to graft the kidney. The liver is a far more difficult organ to remove and replace. The operation can take eight hours or more and involves the painstaking dissection of scores of veins and arteries. It took Starzl the best part of four years to begin finally to crack the problems that he encountered. His clinical programme had begun at the Veterans' Administration Hospital in Denver, Colorado, in March 1963 when he operated on a three-year-old boy suffering from biliary atresia, an incurable congenital defect of the liver. The child bled to death. He made four more unsuccessful attempts in 1963, and had to abandon the technique.

'A pall settled over the liver programme,' says Starzl, 'and no more patients were entered for more than three years. It was the beginning of a self-imposed moratorium.'[65]

Starzl went back to the experimental laboratory to solve the daunting surgical and immunological problems. In 1967, after moving to the University of Pittsburgh, he tried again, this time using the two mainstream anti-rejection drugs, Imuran and Prednisone, in combination with a serum derived from horses called ALG (antilymphocyte globulin). Three of his first seven patients lived for more than a year with their transplanted livers, one surviving for two and a half years. These were the first successful liver transplants, a therapy that today regularly saves thousands of lives each year.

Just as Starzl was beginning to solve the problems of liver transplantation, surgeons in America, Britain and South Africa were preparing themselves for transplant surgery's biggest battle: the attempt to transplant the human heart. Surgically, this was not a difficult operation, but the mystique that surrounds the heart, its ages-old link with love, affection and death, was a sure guarantee that whoever first transplanted it would be destined for immortality. Plenty of ambitious cardiac surgeons were willing to try, but by 1970, their efforts had dragged transplantation down into its darkest hour.

'This was the only example I know in the growth of transplant science,' says Francis Moore, 'where people kind of lost their judgement. In simple phraseology, they went nuts, they went crazy.'

3

The Man with the Golden Hands

It was a warm summer's day in Cape Town, South Africa, when Denise Darvall set off in her new car to see some family friends. Her younger brother, Keith, was sitting beside her. Their parents, Myrtle and Edward, were in the back seats. It was Saturday 2 December 1967 and the Darvalls were in a fine mood. Denise had been teaching Keith to play the theme from the *Doctor Zhivago* movie on the piano, which they were all singing as they drove down Main Road on their way out of the city.

'My wife wanted a cake for our friends,' explained Edward Darvall, 'so we stopped opposite that bakery at Salt River. She got out with Denise and because she liked the cream doughnuts they make at that bakery I told her to get some of them too. "No," she said. "We'll just get the cake – won't be a minute." '[1]

Denise and Myrtle never returned. As they walked back to the car carrying the cake they had just bought from the Wrensch Town Bakery, a lorry blocked their view of the busy road. Perhaps mother and daughter were deep in conversation. Perhaps they just forgot to look before crossing. We will never know why but they were oblivious to the white car that was speeding towards them as they walked past the parked truck and stepped out into the road.

'We heard a thud and a bang and a screech of tyres,' said Edward. 'Keith turned round. "Dad!" he shouted. "It's Mom and Denise!" '[2]

The two women were knocked right across the road. Edward and Keith got out of their car and raced to the scene. 'I saw them lying in the road and everything seemed to go black in front of me,' Edward continued. 'I next found myself sitting down on the sidewalk. Then all of a sudden it came back to me, but there were so many people I couldn't get near my wife. She looked so still and not moving at all that I was suddenly scared she was hurt real bad.'[3]

Fifty-two-year-old Myrtle was dead, killed instantly by the impact. Her daughter had suffered terrible head injuries: blood was pouring from her nose, ears and mouth but she was breathing and her heart still beating when a doctor and an ambulance arrived at the roadside.

At precisely the same time as the Darvalls had been driving up Main Road, Ann Washkansky was with her sister-in-law saying farewell to her husband, Louis, in Ward A1 at Groote Schuur Hospital. Louis was dying. Two major heart-attacks had destroyed so much of the muscle of the pump that had kept him alive for the past fifty-three years that it had hardly the strength to keep the blood moving round his body. 'He couldn't breathe. He couldn't turn without puffing. He couldn't do a thing for himself,' recalls Georgie Declerk, one of the nurses who were Louis's lifeline during the three weeks he had been lying in hospital. 'He was blue. His body was bloated. His legs were draining fluid. He was a very sick man – a very, very sick man indeed. He didn't have long to live.'

Ann kissed her husband goodbye, walked down to her car and drove away from the hospital. Groote Schuur lies on the lower slopes of Table Mountain, the 3500-feet-high dramatic backdrop to Cape Town. A steep drive leads down from the hospital to traffic lights at its junction with Main Road – the very same Main Road on which Denise Darvall was now lying, less than a mile away, unconscious and surrounded by a crowd of curious onlookers. Ann Washkansky turned left at the lights and began the drive back into the city. It took only a minute to reach the site of the accident. She turned to her sister-in-law Grace Sklar. 'We saw this enormous crowd and I said: "Oh, my God, there's been an accident, there's a woman in the road." Grace said to me: "There are two women." When we slowed down we saw one of them was covered. I wondered what she looked like and if I knew her. You never know how lucky you are sometimes. Pity that poor woman.'[4]

Once again fate had conjured up an improbable circumstance. By chance the paths of two families had crossed just a matter of hours before their lives and deaths were to be inextricably linked by medical science. Ann Washkansky's sighting that day of the stricken Denise Darvall was the prelude to the start of a new era in medicine that would revolutionize our understanding of death, transform our centuries-old appreciation of the human heart, bring transplant surgery into the deepest controversy and transform the life of an unknown cardiac surgeon.

Forty-five-year-old Dr Christiaan Barnard was one of the best surgeons in Groote Schuur Hospital but he wasn't the easiest of men to work with. 'When he came into the operating theatre, everyone would change into top gear,' says Dene Friedmann, one of the nurses who worked with him. 'He was an absolute perfectionist . . . and was likely to shout and scream during an operation when he was feeling a bit nervous, so everything had to be absolutely perfect otherwise you knew that you would be in for it. . . . But we all had great respect for him, great admiration and great trust in him as a leader and a surgeon.'

Barnard was a pioneer. He had introduced a surgical treatment for intestinal atresia, a once-fatal interruption of the blood supply to the bowel. He had found a technique that significantly improved the chances of 'blue' babies – children born with the main blood vessels of the heart joined to the wrong sides of the organ. And he'd also developed a heart valve to help prevent deaths from Ebstein's anomaly, another childhood cardiac killer. 'Let me be honest,' he writes. 'I've always been a bad loser. I've always wanted to be the best. . . . And after all, was that so bad? If I *was* the best it meant I'd be giving my patient the best too. Many in the medical profession will disagree and say their first concern is for their patient. A noble sentiment perhaps – but nonsense. A doctor, like anyone else from the playing field to the pulpit, wants, above all, to satisfy his own ambition and ego. It's perfectly human and doctors are, after all, only human.'[5]

The heart is a relatively simple organ – a muscle that pumps blood round the body – and the surgery required to transplant it is relatively straightforward. Rejection was the main obstacle but, with increasing numbers of patients living with trans-planted kidneys, this did not seem a major hurdle to cardiac surgeons, who wanted to extend the frontiers of spare-part surgery.

Barnard entered the transplant arena in 1966 by spending three months at the Medical College of Virginia in America helping David Hume to transplant kidneys.[6] On his return to Cape Town, he did one himself. It was a success: his patient lived for twenty-three years on the grafted organ. Learning how to transplant kidneys, says Barnard, 'played a tremendous part in my decision to do a heart transplant, because I realized . . . that you could take a vital organ from a non-related person and transplant it, and you had the drugs that could control rejection to such an extent that that organ could survive for quite a long period of time.'

Barnard first thought about transplanting a human heart in the early 1960s and had taken the first step of turning the dream into a reality in the experimental animal laboratories at Groote Schuur Hospital. In 1963 he took the heart from a dog's chest and grafted it into a second animal. By the autumn of 1967 his team of surgeons had done nearly fifty of these experimental transplants. Barnard didn't use drugs to keep his transplanted animals alive for long periods; other surgeons, he felt, had already done this work. His only aim was to perfect the surgical technique of heart transplantation and by October 1967 he felt ready to try it on a person. Professor Velva 'Val' Schrire was in charge of the hospital's cardiac unit and the only person who could provide him with a suitable patient and Barnard recalls Schrire's hostility when he first raised the idea with him.

'Your dogs don't live very long,' Schrire told him. 'You should get longer survivors before you try this.' Barnard told him that he hadn't been trying for long-term survival in dogs: 'I can't nurse a dog like a human being,' he said. 'I can't handle a dog on immuno-suppressive drugs as I can a human being.' Schrire thought Barnard was trying to run before he could walk: 'We have first to consider all the risks,' he told him. But Barnard was not to be put off. 'What risks are you talking about?' he asked Schrire angrily. 'We're preparing to do this on a patient with irreversible disease, who is beyond hope of recovery and who has only a few days or hours of life. You call that a risk?' Schrire stood his ground. 'Some people will,' he said. Barnard kept up the pressure. 'Not the man who's about to die – and you know it, Val. He will beg you for it. He'll beg you for the chance. Because that's what it means to him – a chance, not a risk.'[7] At the end of a difficult discussion, the best Barnard could get was a promise from Schrire that he would think about it.

After several weeks of Barnard's persistent badgering, Schrire finally granted the surgeon his wish. He had a patient, Louis Washkansky, a businessman in the last stages of heart failure for whom all other treatments had failed, and he was now willing to show Barnard the green light. But there was one condition: Schrire insisted that the donor of the world's first human heart transplant be white, as well as the recipient.

No such concerns had hampered the choice of Barnard's first kidney transplant in which the recipient was white and the donor black. But Schrire had a clear understanding that the eyes of the world would turn in their direction as soon as news of the heart transplant leaked out. This was, after all, a highly experimental treatment and there was no sense in giving reporters the chance of making them scapegoats for South African racism. 'Those were the days of apartheid,' says Barnard, 'and we were afraid that the world would say: "Look. You see! They use black people and black donors. They experiment on them. That's why they could do the first transplant." So we took those precautions even though they had no medical basis. We were trying to shield ourselves against criticism.'

The news of Barnard's plan was broken to Louis Washkansky by his consultant physician Barry Kaplan. 'I said to him: "Louis, something may be able to be done for you, but it entails a tremendous gamble,"' Kaplan recalls. ' "It is such a gamble you may not come out of it alive." So he says to me: "What is it?" I said: "Professor Schrire said to me that there was a possibility they might be able to transplant somebody's heart into you." He sort of looked at me and said: "If that's the only chance, I'll take it." So I said: "Louis, don't you want to think about it? Don't you want to discuss it with Ann?" He said: "No. No. There's nothing to think about. I can't go on living like this." '[8]

A dying man clutched at the only straw he was offered. It didn't matter to Louis what the treatment was as long as it contained a glimmer of hope for the future. But the idea of transplanting a human heart was such a radical notion in 1967 that Ann Washkansky could not comprehend what Louis was saying when he told her what Barnard was planning. 'I said to him: "Do you mean he's going to put a valve in?" He said: "No, not a valve" and he swore. He said: "A heart! He's going to put a heart in!" And my sister-in-law said to me: "Just humour him. Don't argue with him. If he says a heart, let it be a heart, you know." But we really didn't believe him . . . And then Barnard called me in and I thought to myself: What is this man doing? I said: "You mean, Professor Barnard, you've got to wait for somebody to die?" So he says that's more or less what it is . . . and, of course, that haunted me for months. I got to the stage where I used to look in the newspapers to see if somebody had died or if somebody's heart had been taken . . . It was very traumatic for the family.'

Ann Washkansky was unable to reconcile herself to the idea: it was such an alien concept – the removal of her husband's heart, the seat of his soul, and its replacement with the heart of a stranger. She knew this represented Louis's only chance of survival but she did her best to dissuade him from going ahead. 'I realized they would have to kill Louis, take his heart out, then put somebody else's heart in, not knowing whether it was going to work at all,' she says. 'And that I could not live with – I could not sign for that . . . I mean it was my husband and I would sort of put him to death . . . I tried very hard to stop him from having it done because of that reason but he wouldn't hear of it. He couldn't wait to have it done and he really thought this man was a genius . . . He used to refer to Barnard as the Man with the Golden Hands. He used to say it in Yiddish. He looked upon him as a god.'

Barnard set up a special transplant team, ready to react at any hour of the day or night to the arrival of a suitable donor in the hospital. They didn't have long to wait. Barely a month after

Louis Washkansky had decided that the uncertainty of a successful transplant was preferable to the painful certainty of his failing heart, Denise Darvall was rushed, near to death, into Groote Schuur Hospital. Edward Darvall caught a glimpse of his daughter as she was wheeled through a corridor surrounded by a team of doctors frantically trying to save her life. 'When I saw that, it was another kick in the stomach,' he recalls. 'They'd put a tube in her nose and a doctor was pumping air into her with a black bag while they moved her along on a stretcher with wheels.'[9]

The doctors were fighting a losing battle. An X-ray of her head revealed why: the impact had fractured Denise's skull in two places, one break extending across the base to both ears, the other into her nose. A series of tests showed she had no hope of regaining consciousness. Her eyes were fixed and dilated, she did not react to pain, she had no reflexes and there was no electrical activity coming from her brain. Without the drugs, blood transfusions and the artificial respirator that was making her breathe, her heartbeat would cease. Denise Darvall's brain was dead, but her body was being kept alive by modern technology.

Dr Peter Rose-Innes, the hospital's senior neurosurgeon, had seen many patients like this: human bodies kept alive only by machinery. He had long ago concluded that there was no point in prolonging such lives. Yet in 1967 this, also, was a revolutionary notion. Since time immemorial, the heartbeat had marked the frontier between life and death. The presence of a pulse signified hope, its absence despair. But the development of sophisticated drugs and machinery that could keep patients' bodies functioning long after they had lost any hope of independent existence made it imperative to find a new definition of death. Rose-Innes was in the forefront of the search. 'We were developing the idea of a point of death that could be recognized when the whole brain had stopped functioning permanently while the heart continued to beat,' he says. 'We would diagnose with great care the point at which we were sure the brain was permanently and irrevocably dead and then we would stop using extraordinary means of supporting the patient's heart action.'

Rose-Innes spent several minutes in Denise Darvall's room double-checking the tests to make sure there was no change in the patient's condition. Then he took the first step on a road that revolutionized our understanding of the ending of life and paved the way for the world's first heart transplant. He declared Denise Darvall dead – even though her heart was still beating. It was a highly controversial judgement in a world in which the heart had long had such a central role in the definition of death. By deciding that Denise Darvall would never again regain consciousness and then keeping her body alive until her heart could be removed and transplanted, Rose-Innes was flying in the face of long-established tradition. He had started a process that would knock the heart off the pedestal it had occupied for so long. No longer would it be the final arbiter in the ending of human life: the search for a pulse would be replaced by the search for activity in the brain. A new definition of death – the death of the brain – would become the accepted way of determining the ending of life.

'It was a very revolutionary idea and doctors are, on the whole, relatively conservative, particularly in matters like this,' says Peter Rose-Innes. 'It was difficult. Even though one had thought about it extensively theoretically, to do something like that is always stressful. One wonders whether there was some aspect that one hadn't thought about. But in the event . . . I was quite sure it was the correct thing to do.'

South African legislation gave Rose-Innes great latitude to introduce this new concept of death. 'Our lawyers stated that a patient could be considered a donor once two doctors, one being qualified for more than five years, declared that an individual is dead,' explained Christiaan Barnard. 'It did not state what criteria the doctors had to use. They left that to the medical profession. So we were able to use brain-death as the moment of death to remove the heart.'

Denise Darvall had ceased to live and was now a potential organ donor. A doctor approached Edward Darvall to ask his permission to use Denise's heart to save Louis Washkansky's life. 'We can't save your daughter, her injuries are too bad,' he said. 'But we have a man in the hospital here and we can save his life if you give us permission to use your daughter's heart.'[10]

Edward Darvall took four minutes to make up his mind. His decision turned Denise Darvall's tragedy into Louis Washkansky's opportunity. 'If they could take my daughter's heart or kidney and put it into someone else, it was better to do that than let it die with her,' he recalled. 'I could never have lived with myself if I hadn't done that. Maybe I would have been haunted by her voice asking me: "Why, Daddy, why didn't you do it? Why didn't you want to help that man to live?" '[11]

In the early hours of 3 December 1967, Louis Washkansky lay in the centre of an operating theatre at Groote Schuur Hospital, his ribcage sawn in half and held open by metal clamps. In the centre of his chest his diseased and oversized heart struggled to keep its owner alive.

'The first I knew about it, he was already in the operating theatre,' Ann Washkansky remembers. 'So I didn't have a chance to even say goodbye to him. I asked them if I could come through and they said no, there was no point now because it was going to be a long, long operation. Oh, it was the longest night of my life. I would never have got through it without the family and friends around me, none of whom ever expected him to get through this anyway . . . We just didn't expect it to work.'

Two small rooms, where instruments were sterilized and surgeons scrubbed their hands, separated the operating theatre in which Louis Washkansky lay from the one containing the body of Denise Darvall. Fourteen doctors, nurses and technicians were preparing Washkansky for his historic operation while a second surgical team was getting ready to open Denise's chest. Christiaan Barnard was in charge of both operations: he would perform the most crucial parts of the transplant in removing Denise's heart and sewing it into Washkansky's body. But before he began he faced an acute dilemma. Should he open her chest while her heart was still beating to ensure the organ was as fresh as possible when removed from her body? He possessed a death certificate, the legal authority he needed to do this, and by doing so he would certainly maximize Louis Washkansky's chances of recovery. But a beating human heart had never been removed in this way before. It was a deeply felt moral issue: most doctors felt that death only happened when the heart stopped. Should he, therefore, bow to tradition, switch off the ventilator and permit the heart to stop beating naturally before making the first incision? It could take ten or fifteen minutes for this to occur during which the lack of oxygen might seriously damage the heart's muscle. It was a fraught moment. Barnard says that he decided to be cautious, allowing the heart to stop naturally – even though the donor had been declared brain-dead and he risked damaging the heart in the process. 'I did not want to touch this girl until she was conventionally dead – a corpse,' he wrote in his autobiography. 'Brain-death had already been established, but I felt we could not put a knife into her until she was truly a cadaver.'[12] Today he points to his fear of the consequences to justify a decision that potentially placed Louis Washkansky at greater risk. 'If I opened her chest while the heart was still beating the world would criticize it and say: "Look, you're not allowed to do that. You have to wait until the heart stops beating because that's the moment of death." I didn't consider that the moment of death, but because the cessation of heart-beat was an accepted criterion of death, I didn't want to expose myself to that criticism.'

Barnard says that only when the respirator had been switched off and oxygen starvation had finally stopped Darvall's heartbeat, did he instruct his surgical team to begin the task of cutting through her ribcage. He then walked back to the theatre where Louis Washkansky was lying deeply unconscious, his blood supply ready to be linked up to a heart-lung machine. This was a crucial piece of equipment: without the ability to re-route the blood away from the heart, keeping it artificially oxygenated and flowing through a patient's arteries and veins, neither heart transplantation nor most forms of open-heart surgery would be possible. Louis Washkansky's life depended on the machine's efficient functioning, and a wave of near panic spread through the operating theatre when Barnard told a nurse to clamp a tube carrying Washkansky's blood without first turning off the machine. It was such a serious error that it nearly cost the patient his life. 'For some reason I said, clamp the line. . . . So the nursing sister clamped the line with the heart-lung machine still pumping. It built up such pressure that it disconnected the tube and blood was spurting all over the machine . . .'

Barnard and his technicians worked feverishly to remove the air bubbles from the heart-lung machine and restore their patient's circulation. They only had a few minutes before the lack of oxygen-rich blood to his brain would plunge Washkansky into the same vegetative state as the unfortunate Denise Darvall. 'If I didn't have things worked out how to handle the situation it could have caused the death of Louis Washkansky before we even did the transplant,' says Barnard.

The operation went smoothly after this initial disaster. Barnard returned to Denise Darvall's body, severed the major blood vessels connecting her heart to her chest and carried it back into the first operating theatre. With Louis Washkansky safely back on the heart-lung machine, he began to remove his patient's diseased heart. The moment he took it out is burned into his memory. 'I've often seen the inside of a chest but I've never seen a human being who was actually alive without a heart inside his chest. And I realized at that stage that I was doing something different. I'd never done this before. I realized that I had to put a heart back there and I had to get that heart to start working again if I wanted to get my patient to survive and recover. It was an eerie feeling. It was something that I've never experienced before in my life.'

The disturbing void in the middle of Louis Washkansky's chest was quickly filled. Denise Darvall's small, healthy heart was sewn into the cavity, the stumps of the blood vessels that once united it with its former owner were securely joined to their counterparts in its new home. Barnard checked the joins to make sure they were leakproof, removed the clamps and allowed blood to enter the heart.

The heart muscle twitched back to life as soon as the blood entered its empty chambers. But it was fibrillating – beating in an uncoordinated and uncontrolled manner. To restore a regular heartbeat, the surgeon picked up two metal paddles, placed one on either side of Washkansky's new heart, and passed an electric current through the muscle. Washkansky's body jerked as the electricity flowed through his body. Dene Friedmann, who was in the theatre, remembers the moment. 'Although they had the utmost confidence in Professor Barnard, it had never been done before in a human being. We were all worried – was that heart going to start beating? – and so for that few seconds there was absolute quietness and . . . the next thing the heart started beating and it was absolutely wonderful. The jubilation. Everybody was smiling. It was really a superb moment.'

The spiky tracing on the electrocardiograph now showed a reassuringly regular rise and fall. The new heart was beating normally. But the battle wasn't quite over. There was one more hurdle to cross: would Washkansky's new heart support his circulation once the heart-lung machine was switched off? This was the final test of the viability of the transplant and the tension in the operating theatre rose several notches again as Barnard gave the order to switch off the machine. The heart struggled as it lost support and Barnard had to switch the machine back on. He let it rest and tried again. Once again the heart began to fail. Anxiety filled the atmosphere as he tried a third time.

'When the heart-lung machine stopped for a third time,' says Barnard, 'the doctor who gave the anaesthetic called out the pressures – and all the pressures showed it was carrying the circulation. . . . It was like we were in darkness and all of a sudden a bright light came on in the operating room and I then stretched my hand across to my first assistant and I said to him: "It's going to work."'

Barnard had taken a deliberately low-key approach to the transplant. The press had not been told about the operation before it took place. There wasn't even a hospital photographer to record the event for posterity. The story didn't appear until a few hours after Louis Washkansky was wheeled out of the theatre, his new heart beating soundly inside his chest. Suddenly, the world's first human heart transplant was headline news all over the world. Not in their wildest dreams had Christiaan Barnard and his team imagined they would become the focus of the media circus that now laid siege to Groote Schuur Hospital.

'There were press and photographers everywhere,' recalls Dene

Friedmann. 'I think they were photographing everybody in sight. You could hardly move in the corridors ... Nobody ever expected it to hit the media like it did and when we saw the papers the next morning with these big headlines, "Human Heart Transplant Performed in Cape Town" we were really very proud.'

But the media invasion wasn't entirely good news as far as the surgical team at the hospital was concerned. 'It just became impossible to work,' says Barnard, 'because of the demands put on me by the media. I recognized what they wanted but I don't think they recognized that I had to have time to look after my patients, to do my surgery. I couldn't spend all my time answering questions and appearing in front of cameras. . . . It really amazed me that there was so much controversy, so much criticism, so much praise, so much excitement about the operation. It was not that great an event – certainly not in the history of medicine.'

On a strictly surgical level, Barnard might be right: the operation to replace Washkansky's heart was not technically difficult. What made it such a media feast was the special place reserved for the heart in the human psyche: when we think about love and affection we think about the organ that's beating inside our chests. It is not, after all, the kidney or the liver that Tony Bennett left in San Francisco. Our deep emotional attachment to this humble organ guaranteed that whoever first swapped a new heart for an old would earn a secure place in history, and when it turned out to be an unknown surgeon in a country better known for racism and brutality than cardiac surgery, the world beat a path to Groote Schuur Hospital. It was the first good news story to come out of South Africa for years. The country that had become an international pariah was suddenly back in favour and foreign accolades were eagerly reprinted in the *Cape Times*. According to the paper, the *Washington Daily News* trumpeted the transplant as 'another frontier conquered – a frontier no less important and far more immediate than the stars'. The *New York Daily News*, meanwhile, was apparently describing Barnard's feat as a 'marvellous story', which gave the feeling that medical progress 'has only just got off to a good beginning'. The head of the Central Red Cross Hospital in Spain was also quoted. He called the transplant 'formidable and sensational . . . even if the patient was lost, the operation constitutes a great achievement'.[13] Christiaan Barnard won the praise and South Africans basked in the limelight.

But much of the research into heart transplants had not been done by Barnard. When the story of his pioneering operation finally surfaced, there were many astonished faces. Three had more reason to be surprised than most: three surgeons who did their best to beat Barnard to the finishing post but who were delayed by the ethical concerns raised by heart transplantation.

The first was Donald Longmore, an English physician and experimental surgeon working at the National Heart Hospital in London. A nurse broke the news to him. 'Well, one has to admit that there was a little twinge of disappointment,' he says. 'But, on the other hand, I was so thrilled that it had happened, and that really far outweighed any personal disappointments . . . I hoped and prayed that it would go well so that we'd be allowed to go ahead and all the opposition would be squashed.'

If Longmore had had his way, the first team to transplant a human heart would have been in London, not Cape Town. He had long recognized that the heart was logically the next organ to be transplanted after the kidney and the liver. But he had reckoned without the conservative nature of the British medical profession and the British public, who thought it couldn't – or even shouldn't – be transplanted, as he found out one day when giving a fund-raising speech. 'I said: "Hands up anybody here who would be prepared to have a kidney transplant." All the hands went up. "Hands up those who would be prepared to have a liver transplant." Quite a lot of hands went up. "Hands up those who would be prepared to have a heart or a heart-lung transplant." There were a few sort of timorous hands going half-way up and then they looked up and pulled them down again. Now why on earth was that? Well, there were two reasons, I think. First of all, the feeling that the heart is mythically to do with the soul and the spirit and that it was wrong, and also the feeling that if you took a beating heart out of somebody, they were actually alive when you took it out.'

The feelings Christiaan Barnard had wrestled with before removing Denise Darvall's heart were widespread. They might be rooted in emotion and medical ignorance but they were real stumbling blocks to the desire to transplant the human heart. Donald Longmore, however, was an experimental scientist who believed it was the right moment to break with tradition and write a new chapter in the story of transplant surgery. Since 1963, he had spent two or three days a week and many weekends in a basement laboratory at the Royal Veterinary College doing hundreds of experimental animal heart and heart-lung transplant operations. By the mid 1960s he thought he had acquired enough surgical and immunological skills to undertake the world's first human heart transplant. He even had a patient, a milkman called Bill Bradley who had suffered a massive heart-attack and whose heart muscle had been damaged beyond repair. 'He wasn't able to walk very far,' explains his widow Betty. 'On a good day he could walk up the garden, but on a very bad day he had to be shaved. I had to help him in the bath, and I had to wash him. He always had to have oxygen by the side of his bed. He was on pain-killers – lots and lots of tablets I had to give him.'

Bill Bradley was willing to try his luck with a transplant. He had no other choice. Longmore believed it could be done – and told him as much in a letter written in November 1967. What Longmore did not have was the authority to perform one on his own. He was indeed a trained surgeon but because he had decided, some years earlier, to specialize as a physician, he could not now operate on patients. He was convinced that the heart transplant was a feasible operation but he needed to persuade more senior surgical colleagues at the National Heart Hospital. And they didn't want to know. The conservative British medical establishment were anxious to avoid being steam-rollered into heart transplants before the scientific, ethical and legal problems had been fully resolved. In Donald Longmore's eyes, they were scared of taking the first step.

'Well, there was substantial opposition from the medical establishment, both within this hospital and without,' says Longmore. 'And it was based on three things, really. One was lack of knowledge, because they didn't know about the huge amount of research which had been done here. . . . The second thing was a lack of guts. It's easier to say no than to have a go. And the third thing was a lack of vision. Heart surgery, you will remember, was just starting, and people couldn't conceive that it could have advanced from doing simple plumbing and changing valves on to something which is biologically more complex. . . . There was a huge amount of opposition and you have to remember that I was only a young junior surgeon at that time, not in a position to force these things through.'

Bill Bradley never had his heart transplant. About eighteen months after Donald Longmore suggested that this was his only hope, he had another heart-attack and died. 'I think he was cheated out of life,' says his son Leslie. 'He'd been in pain for so long, he'd waited so long for this but it hadn't happened. . . . You couldn't talk to him without him discussing it, saying: "I'm ready, I'm just waiting for it. I want the improvements. I want to live a life again. And if they give me three or five years, I will be very happy, very happy indeed." I just thought he was cheated.'

'I agree with them,' says Donald Longmore. 'Totally. But not for malicious reasons or anything like that – just ignorant gutless people which happens so often in life. It wasn't even resources which were short. It was the opportunity.'

The second of the three surprised surgeons was Dr Norman Shumway, a cardiac surgeon at Stanford University Medical Centre, near San Francisco in California. Shumway had done more experimental work on heart transplantation than anyone else. He had been swapping hearts between dogs in the Medical Centre's laboratories since 1959. By 1967 he had published more than twenty academic papers on the surgical technique and the immunological aftercare of his transplanted animals. Some of his dogs lived for several months after their operations. A few survived for as long as a year. It wasn't spectacular but several months before Barnard took the plunge, Shumway had reached the conclusion that it was time to try the operation on a patient. 'Survival of dogs after any kind of cardiac surgery is different from people,' explains Shumway. 'The human is the king of the jungle – there's no question about it: much stronger . . . and we had as good survival in our animals as anybody had in kidney or liver transplantation in animals.'

There were several patients in the Medical Centre whose heart problems were so severe that only a transplant might save their lives. What Shumway needed was a suitable donor, an individual declared brain-dead whose heart could be kept beating until it was ready to be transplanted. Here, Shumway ran into a serious legal hurdle. In America in 1967 there was no ambiguity about the definition of death: the legal dictionary stated clearly that life ended when, among other things, the heart stopped beating and the blood circulation ceased. Shumway dismissively calls this the 'boy-scout' definition of death, but it was widely accepted among the American medical profession. 'Brain-death' was a much more controversial idea in America than it was in South Africa. It had the potential to place doctors on the wrong side of the law and Shumway was unable to find a neurosurgeon willing to declare anyone dead until their heart had ceased beating. 'We had to have the co-operation of people who were knowledgeable in making the diagnosis of brain-death and we couldn't get it,' he says. 'They were saying they believed that the death of the individual is the absence of the heartbeat and the circulation. . . . For example, they'd have a brain-dead accident victim on life support and when the patient was brain-dead they would turn off the respirator and walk away. And twenty minutes later when the heart had stopped they would come in and declare the patient dead. . . . Everybody knew about brain-death but it was such a change of tradition that it wasn't easily accepted anywhere. It was almost inevitable that the first transplant would be done in a developing country.'

Shumway was not prepared to risk transplanting a heart that might have been damaged by stopping naturally, so he was unable to get his clinical heart-transplant programme off the ground until he found a private neurosurgeon willing to risk professional disapproval, and even a court summons, by supplying him with a brain-dead donor, which only happened four weeks after Chris Barnard's operation on Louis Washkansky. 'We had no idea he was interested in heart transplantation,' he explains. 'Our people felt that we'd done all the work in the field . . . I think there was no question that, at that time, there was in Chris's mind [the thought] that he'd better do one quickly or we – or somebody else – would.'

Shumway would never admit it himself, but he didn't take the news of Barnard's coup very well. Ed Stinton, a junior surgeon in the Medical Centre at the time, remembers the moment the media caught up with his boss, shortly after he had heard the first report from Groote Schuur Hospital. 'Doctor Shumway was in the habit of making rounds with us,' explains Stinton, 'and then taking us to the cafeteria where he'd buy us coffee and doughnuts. That morning, in contrast to his usual self, he was very, very quiet. One reporter caught up with us in the cafeteria and I remember him being very clipped with him when asked what he thought about it. I think that Dr Shumway was very angry . . . He had devoted more than a decade of his investigational career to this particular procedure and had started moving in all the appropriate directions for the clinical application. For someone like Barnard to come along and basically exploit it in an opportunistic fashion, I think probably made Dr Shumway very angry. He seized that particular opportunity for glory and fame.'

The third despondent surgeon was Adrian Kantrowitz, a cardiac specialist at the Maimonides Medical Centre in Brooklyn, New York. 'I'd been doing heart surgery for many years,' he explains, 'and we would constantly come across patients whose hearts were so damaged that it was . . . hard to conceive of any technique that could repair them to the point where they could have a reasonable life.' He had also spent long hours in the laboratory perfecting the surgical technique of heart transplantation on dogs and trying to overcome the immunological problems. Some of his animals were living for up to a year after their operations. By the summer of 1966, more than a year before Barnard was ready to go ahead, Kantrowitz felt he had gained sufficient experience to try the technique on a patient. He was well aware of the legal and moral problems but he thought he had found a way of overcoming the medical profession's reluctance to move away from the traditional definition of death. He decided to restrict his search for a suitable heart donor to the small number of anencephalitic babies (lacking a brain) born in America each year. The children are badly deformed, the top of their skull is missing and in its place is a bulbous, leathery coating of skin. Usually they live no longer than a few days and Kantrowitz thought that, provided he received permission from the parents, there would be no moral or legal objection to the use of an anencephalitic baby's heart to save the life of another infant.

'They really are born essentially dead, from a human point of view,' he says. 'There is no possibility that such a child could develop into a functioning human being . . . and we knew that a large percentage of these infants had good hearts. So . . . here we felt we could with all conscience use the heart of an infant while it was still beating because this child was dead already – because this child had no brain and there was no possibility of repairing the brain.'

It was not as simple as Kantrowitz had hoped. To transplant the beating heart of an anencephalitic baby, he had to win the agreement of a wide spectrum of medical opinion at Maimonides Medical Centre: from the obstetricians who would be providing the donor child, the paediatricians who would be taking care of the baby after its birth, the cardiologists who could vouch for the health of the donor's heart; and the research committee at the hospital, whose approval was required for such an experimental operation. This was too much to ask in the climate of opinion current in America in the mid 1960s.

Kantrowitz received the hospital's permission to transplant the heart of an anencephalitic baby but his colleagues insisted that he let the infant's heart stop naturally before it was removed. 'They were all very uncomfortable,' he says, 'because we were stepping off into a field which had been totally unexplored and they didn't know that they wouldn't be criticized if they permitted me to use a heart that was still beating. . . . They were concerned that even though I felt that such a child had no possibility of developing . . . they did not want to be part of removing a heart from an individual when it was still beating.'

This was far from an ideal situation – but not an impossible one. It was difficult to transplant a heart that had stopped beating, but Kantrowitz's own laboratory experiments had shown that it could be done. He decided it was worth a try. In June 1966 his chance came when Miller Stevenson was born at the Medical Centre with one side of his heart missing – an incurable and lethal defect. Kantrowitz began to look for a suitable anencephalitic donor by canvassing hospitals around America. He found one 2,600 miles away in Oregon on the west coast.

Rhoda Senz had had no reason to think that the birth of her fourth child would be any different from the last three. She had already had three healthy boys and, although this pregnancy had been uncomfortable, she was as excited as any expectant mother at the prospect of the new arrival. Her husband, Richard, was sitting on a couch outside the delivery room when the baby was born. A doctor brought him the devastating news.

'He described the condition of the baby,' explains Richard, 'the malformation of the head area, and he said there was no way that this child was going to survive . . . I mean they . . . never brought the baby in to the mother as they normally do in a delivery situation. I was pretty well distraught. All I was concerned about was the condition of the baby and the condition of my wife.'

Rhoda had been sedated near the end of the birth. The first she knew of the terrible defect was when Richard came in to tell her that she had given birth to an anencephalitic baby. He also explained the request their doctor had made: that they consider donating the child's heart to save the life of Miller Stevenson. Richard says, 'I was totally open-minded about it after I realized that there was only a short time that this baby was going to live, and I felt that if we could contribute to some other life, why we would be very happy about that and I'm sure that the people on the other end that were going to receive it would be happy also.'

Rhoda needed a little persuading – her maternal instincts cried out to protect Ralph, their baby. But after giving the matter some thought, the reasonableness of the request was clear to her. 'Well, for me,' she says, 'it came down to what can we do to salvage some good from a situation that isn't good. We knew that the usual time of life was only three days and so there wasn't an opportunity for our child to live. So to be able to provide an opportunity for another one, it seemed to me there wasn't a choice. That was something we felt very strongly about and so that was a fairly easy decision for us to make.'

A helicopter flew Rhoda and Richard's baby to Maimonides Medical Centre. By the early evening of the next day he was dying. At 11.45 p.m. on 26 June 1966 he was brought into the operating theatre so that the transplant could take place as soon as he died. Adrian Kantrowitz understood the moral qualms of those who had insisted that the infant be allowed to die naturally, but from the medical point of view, it was a pointless exercise. Ralph Senz had no possibility of life. Miller Stevenson did. By permitting Ralph's heart to stop naturally, it was much more likely that two children would die that night, not one. Kantrowitz wanted Miller to have the best possible chance of survival and thought the best way to ensure this was to bend the rules. He wanted to take out Ralph's heart before it had stopped beating, but he faced a reluctant anaesthetist who insisted that he work by the book. Jordan Haller, then the director of cardiovascular surgery in Kantrowitz's department, remembers the tussle between the two men.

'Our anaesthetist, who was a lovely man, a fine kindly grandfather, kept putting a towel over the head of this terribly deformed human new-born and he said: 'You can't take the heart, Adrian, it's beating, it's alive.' Adrian snatched the towel off and forced everyone to look. It was a terrible sight. A headless, brainless human body, the rest of the baby perfectly formed, but no brain, no upper part of the head above the eyes. And Adrian kept repeating, 'There is no brain, it can't be alive, just because the heart beats and the liver functions and the lungs function, doesn't mean that it's a living being.' And Harry, I remember very well, took the towel back, kindly grandfather that he was and said: 'No, its mother and its father consider it their child, its heart is beating – you're not taking the heart until it stops.' Today there would be no hesitation. These arguments would not occur. . . . It was a tragic circumstance but the parents had bravely donated the organs and we were not allowed to use them.'

While the donor baby was dying in one operating theatre, two-month-old Miller Stevenson was lying next door in another waiting for the chance of life. Kantrowitz had decided not to open Miller's chest until Ralph had died and he had checked the condition of his heart. At 12.21 a.m. on 20 June 1966 Ralph's heart finally stopped beating. As rapidly as he could, Kantrowitz opened the infant's chest.

'It didn't look good,' he recalls. 'It was not beating and even though we tried to stimulate it, it wouldn't contract well. The electrocardiogram looked very poor and we felt that if we now subjected the recipient to an operation which would take us another half-hour before we could implant this heart, that it was unlikely to be successful. So we aborted that effort. . . . I'm sure that if we had taken the donor heart out of the child while it was still beating, an hour or two earlier, then we would have had an excellent chance of having the whole procedure go successfully.'

Just under a month after the death of Rhoda and Richard's son, Miller Stevenson's body abandoned the uphill battle it had fought against the suffocating effects of its defective heart. He died of congestive heart failure.

'Oh, we were all devastated. We were all confused,' remembers Jordan Haller. 'We all felt so many emotions. No one had been this path before. We felt we were doing the right thing. We felt we were condemning the recipient. . . . We had to look forward to what we were going to do to the recipient. What's that infant's future? Without a transplant heart it had none either. So we lost two children. We were all quite shaken for a long time about what is right, morally, ethically.'

Rhoda and Richard Senz were never told the reason why the operation failed. The report they received said quite simply that the operation had not been successful. They were surprised when I explained what had happened, saying that the decision to let their child's heart stop naturally was wrong and wasteful.

'I think they should have taken the heart while it was still beating and made the transplant,' says Richard. 'I feel very strongly about that. If you're going to go into something and be successful, give it all the chances it can to be successful. . . . If they would have called us and asked us we would have made the same decision. . . . We accepted there was no chance for survival in our son so, you know, it isn't a violation of anyone's body.'

Eighteen months later, in November 1967, the birth of another baby boy with a badly deformed heart in the hospital gave Kantrowitz his second chance of doing the world's first heart transplant. The child's mother, Anna Scudero, had already had her fair share of tragedy: she'd lost one of her three sons in a road accident and now disaster had befallen her again with the birth of Jamie. 'I didn't know until maybe a couple of days later that he had a hole in his heart,' she says. 'He was chubby and had beautiful black hair all over . . . They put a sign on his crib: "If you can't do nothing with my heart please do something with my hair." I never held him you know. I seen him but I never held the baby. It was hard – very hard.'

Kantrowitz had already tried, unsuccessfully, to repair the defect, and the baby's health was rapidly deteriorating. He knew that a transplant was the child's only hope, even if he was again prevented from taking out the donor heart before it had stopped beating. Anna Scudero gave her consent. 'When they told me they were thinking of the heart transplant I said: "Look, if I don't do it and something happens to him, I won't forgive myself." So I had to sign.'

A donor was found in Philadelphia, another anencephalitic child. The parents gave their permission and the baby was flown into Maimonides Medical Centre. It was early December 1967. The transplant team had again been mobilized and was preparing itself for the operation.

'We all went home, had a drink, relaxed to get ready for the next day or two when we were planning to do the transplant. And the next morning my daughter came in and said it just came over the radio that some doctor had just done a heart transplant in Africa. So I said: "You're kidding!" And she said: "You don't think I'd kid about something like that?" And so then we listened to the radio and it was true that Dr Chris Barnard had just done his successful transplant at the Groote Schuur Hospital in Cape Town, South Africa . . .' Kantrowitz had been pipped at the post by the unknown cardiac surgeon from Cape Town. He is disarmingly honest about the feeling of frustration that overwhelmed him at the time. 'Sure I was disappointed. I felt I could have been rich and famous if I had done it first,' he jokes. 'So I had to settle for what I had. . . . We would have liked to have done the first successful heart transplant in the world. But we were going to do the first successful heart transplant in the United States – and that's not bad either. At any rate, I cannot say I was not disappointed. I was.'

4

The Knife-edge of Survival

With an efficient new heart pumping blood around his body, Louis Washkansky began to make a remarkable recovery. A ventilator prevented him from talking for a few hours after his pioneering operation, but the transformation in his health was obvious from the moment the tube came out of his throat.

'What felt so different was that he didn't have to battle for breath,' says Sister Georgie Declerk, one of the nurses who took care of Washkansky after his operation. 'He could just breathe. There was a dramatic improvement. He was full of fun. He was sitting up, eating, reading, listening to the radio. Wonderful days – wonderful days. Joking with us, he really was. He was very well. . . . It was really amazing.'

Christiaan Barnard was also taken aback by the rapid improvement of a man who had been hovering at death's door: 'He recovered so quickly. It was amazing to see how he lost all evidence of heart failure. The swelling of his leg disappeared, the swelling of his liver disappeared. His lungs became dry, and he was well, mentally well. . . . So we were very optimistic at the beginning, in the first week or so.'

In 1967 Groote Schuur Hospital did not have a special ward set aside for the intensive care of post-operative patients. So Louis Washkansky lay in a private nursing room that had been adapted for his care and safety. An oxygen tent attached to a metal frame was draped over the bed, on either side of which were electronic monitors to give the medical team early warning of any change in his health. The drugs Washkansky was taking to control rejection left him vulnerable to minor infections, so rigorous hygiene was the order of the day. Before the patient arrived, the room was sterilized with disinfectant. The nursing team had regular throat, nose and rectal swabs to check for dangerous micro-organisms, and anyone who came into the room had to wear sterile clothes. There were no exceptions: Ann Washkansky put on a clean hospital gown, gloves, a hat, overshoes and a paper face mask when she first came to see her husband, three days after his operation. She could hardly believe that he had survived and wasn't sure what to expect when she walked into his room. 'I was very apprehensive because I thought his personality might have changed, not realizing that the heart is not the personality, that your brain makes the person,' she says. 'And I was happy to see he was the same Louis. You know, he really thought he was going to have a wonderful life. . . . He was going to go travelling, he was going to dance, he was going to work and he was going to do everything that he really wanted to do without being ill. He hated being ill.'

The transplant team monitored Washkansky day and night. They analysed his blood, checked his pulse, his urine output and the pressure in the chambers of his heart. They took temperature readings and made delicate adjustments to his anti-rejection drugs. The meticulous care and attention that Christiaan Barnard gave his patients at their bedsides was as much a part of his reputation in the hospital as was his famed skill in the operating theatre. 'I remember when he had a sick patient on his hands he would sometimes sit and nurse the patient himself all night,' recalls Dene Friedmann. 'He wouldn't go home at all – he wouldn't leave the patient's bedside. I would say that he fought like a lion, with everything in his power, and even prayed to God. He did everything he possibly could for that patient's life.'

Barnard knew they were walking a tightrope between infection and rejection. The symptoms of one could be easily mistaken for the other – and the wrong treatment might prove fatal to their patient. He wanted as much warning as possible of trouble on the path ahead. But this was unexplored territory and there were no signposts to guide the way.

For five days, Louis Washkansky made better progress than the medical team at Groote Schuur Hospital – or the rest of the world – dared to hope. On the sixth day after the transplant, Barnard drove into work needing no reminder that this was likely to be a crucial time, but the morning news on his car radio rubbed the message home anyway. 'Today Louis Washkansky enters the most critical phase of his new life,' recounted the news-reader. 'The first attempt of his body to reject the heart of Denise Darvall is expected today or tomorrow . . .'[1]

Barnard went into Washkansky's room and said good morning to his patient, who did not reply.

'How's it going, Louis?' Barnard asked again.

'I've had enough, leave me alone.'

'Enough of what?'

'They're killing me. I can't sleep, I can't eat, I can't do anything. They're at me all the time with pins and needles, pins and needles . . . all day and all night. It's driving me crazy.'[2]

This was the first sign of bad temper Barnard had seen in Washkansky since the operation. He sensed that something was wrong – and the medical charts confirmed his fears. There was a marked voltage drop in the electrical output of the heart, a possible sign that his body was rejecting the new organ. More bad news was to follow: the hospital's bacteriologist, who had been taking swabs from various parts of Washkansky's body to check for micro-organisms, told Barnard he had found a particularly dangerous one, the bacterium Klebsiella, in his nostrils, mouth and rectum.

Barnard faced a difficult dilemma: if he treated Washkansky for rejection by increasing the dose of immuno-suppressive drugs, he would further lower his patient's resistance to infection and risk the bacterium getting out of control. But if the heart was being rejected and he gave him only a strong antibiotic to kill the germ, he would be signing his patient's death warrant. The transplant team was groping in the dark. There was no body of clinical experience on which they could lean. For the moment, they decided to sit on the fence, giving antibiotics to knock out the infection and a strong dose of drugs to combat rejection.[3]

It seemed to be the right decision. Louis Washkansky's irritability vanished and the next four days were good humoured and optimistic. But on the eleventh day after his operation, Washkansky awoke with severe pains in his gut. On the twelfth, when he was due to meet a cabinet minister, be photographed by *Stern* magazine and interviewed by the BBC and CBS, he developed a pain in his left shoulder and became increasingly irritable and tired. The visits were cut short. On the thirteenth day the pains grew worse. He experienced difficulty in breathing and an X-ray showed disturbing shadows in his lungs. Barnard's uncertainties grew by the hour. His patient could be suffering from pneumonia – but the medical team had been unable to find any bacteria in his lungs. Perhaps the shadows had been caused by a blood clot that had obstructed the blood supply and killed part of the lungs. There was a third possibility: were the lung shadows a sign of rejection, a condition then called 'transplant lung'? Treatments existed for each condition: antibiotics or other drugs to kill the bacteria; heparin to prevent further blood-clotting; steroids to combat transplant lung. Louis Washkansky's condition was deteriorating rapidly and the margin for error was exceptionally fine: if they treated for one complaint and it turned out to be another, their patient was doomed. There was little time for debate. By the fifteenth day Washkansky was gasping for air, the pain in his chest had spread to his arms and was so severe he was hardly able to move. Spotty patches appeared on his legs – a sure sign of circulatory failure. Washkansky was sliding into oblivion and the transplant team was hopelessly split on what course to take.

Barnard then took a decision he now regrets. He told his team to increase the dose of Imuran and Prednisone and also to begin injecting Washkansky with hydrocortisone. He had decided to treat his patient for transplant lung. Only later did he discover that Washkansky was succumbing to a virulent infection. The wrong diagnosis was the beginning of the end for his patient.

'We made the biggest mistake there,' says Barnard. 'I increased the drugs that stop rejection and therefore made it much worse for him to fight the infection that he had in his lungs . . . I think that if we were able to establish the organisms[4] that were present in his lungs at that stage, and what drug they were sensitive to, and we started treating him straight at that point, I think he would have recovered.'

Sixteen days after his transplant, Washkansky's breathing became so laboured that Barnard had no choice but to place him on a ventilator.

The closing days of Louis's life were a nightmare for Ann Washkansky. Her husband was now public property, her distress no longer a private affair. 'Everything was exposed in the papers,' she says. 'And what I didn't read I was phoned up to read. The reporters would ring me: "Did I see that my husband wasn't well?" That was the first I got to know about it anyway. They hounded me until I did know. That's the one aspect of the press that I found very distasteful.'

On the last day of his life, the anaesthetist disconnected the ventilator and began to force oxygen into Washkansky's chest by hand, a last-ditch attempt to prevent the patient from drowning in the fluid filling his lungs.

'I suppose really I knew he was not going to make it,' says Georgie Declerk. 'I think he himself also knew he wasn't going to make it then. Though he never said anything, you know, "This is it" or "It's over." But it was very sad. We had so much hope that he'd make it. And he didn't.'

Louis Washkansky's fight for life ended on 21 December, eighteen days after he received his new heart.

'I was completely destroyed that morning,' Christiaan Barnard says. 'I stood on that balcony in the hospital as the sun was coming up and he died . . . I was totally destroyed. I went down to my office and I lay on the couch there and one of my black laboratory assistants came in and saw I was crying and he didn't know what to say. He just said to me: "Professor, you're working too hard." '

Louis Washkansky was dead but a new life was about to begin for the man who had stuck his neck out to perform the world's first heart transplant. Christiaan Barnard, an obscure cardiac surgeon from Cape Town, would soon be as famous as the Beatles. The operation had failed, but Barnard had succeeded in breaking a taboo: he'd taken an organ that many people thought couldn't, or shouldn't, be touched, and sewn it into another person. Never mind that the gift of life had only lasted eighteen days – he was a pioneer whose journey into unknown territory was every bit as significant as that of Edmund Hillary and Tenzing Norgay, the first men to climb Mount Everest, or Neil Armstrong, the American astronaut, who would soon take the first steps on the moon. There was a fairy-tale quality to the events that overtook Barnard in the months following the operation on Louis Washkansky. The man whose family had been so poor that they couldn't afford to buy him shoes as a boy was now courted by presidents, royalty and the international press corps. While Ann Washkansky was shedding tears for Louis at his funeral in Cape Town, Christiaan Barnard was on his way to a TV studio in Washington DC to make an appearance on the prestigious CBS *Face the Nation* show. He and his wife Louwtjie had been booked into the Presidential suite at the Washington Hilton Hotel where, Barnard wryly reflected at the time, his month's salary would hardly cover the costs of the wine, let alone the room. Overnight his life was transformed.

'I mean here's a little boy who was born in the Karoo,[5] had a very humble beginning, and then worked in a southern part of South Africa where very little that you do is recognized – and all of a sudden I'm a celebrity,' he says. 'Everybody wants to talk to me, everyone wants to meet me. I get invitations left, right and centre. It was exciting. It was very exciting. I do admit that . . . sometimes I lost my balance because I loved the exposure so much.'

Barnard joined the jet set. Over the next year or two he travelled to many different countries to tell the story of the first heart transplant. He became South Africa's most valued ambassador. He flew to America to meet the President, Lyndon B. Johnson; he travelled to Monaco to see Prince Rainier and Princess Grace; he went to Germany, Brazil, England, Spain, Peru, Iran and Italy, where he was granted an audience with the Pope.

'I once went to Rome,' he recalls, 'and a friend of mine was with me and as the plane was taxiing up to the terminal you could just see thousands of people. And I said, "What's happening there?" And he says, "I don't know." So the plane stopped, and they told me not to get out. And then he went out and he came back and said, "Chris, those thousands of people are there to see you, to wait for you, just to touch you." It was really an unbelievable experience. I think at one stage I was probably one of the most popular people in the world.'

He was certainly popular with the South African government whose image he was boosting – unwittingly, perhaps – with every foreign TV appearance. The municipal authorities in Cape Town honoured him with the freedom of the city and the central government presented him with the country's highest award, the Hendrik Verwoerd Medal.

But in one place Christiaan Barnard was becoming increasingly unpopular. His home. Louwtjie sometimes accompanied him on his whirlwind foreign tours but she found her husband's new-found status as a superstar an increasing burden. 'Oh, in the beginning, I also thought it was wonderful to go on these trips,' she says, 'but in the end I got sick and tired of it, you know. Like I once said, we're not the Beatles. Or when people rush up to tear your coat buttons off and things, I thought: "No. This is terrible. I just want to be me. I don't want to be public property." I didn't know there was a world like that. You know, I saw it on film but it didn't really interest me. I kept on thinking: "What am I doing here? Shouldn't I be at home looking after my children . . . than with this man who did the operation?" '

The Barnards' marriage had never been easy. There had been rows long before Christiaan became a figure on the world stage, but the endless foreign tours, the media demands, the adulation and the honours placed even more strain on their fragile relationship. 'He was definitely affected,' says Louwtjie, 'because he was a guy that hardly possessed a suit and then suddenly he came home with the most wonderful clothes and stood in front of the mirror and looked at himself. He just changed. He just wasn't Chris any more. There was just this man inside him that's now famous and fame is a terrible thing. You know there wasn't this nice gentle guy any more, who could smile and laugh. He did it all for the public and for the people out there.' The fame and the publicity, Louwtjie Barnard felt, were driving a wedge between her husband and his children – and between her and her friends.

But far worse than this were the other women in her husband's life. The man who had transplanted the first human heart suddenly realized he had no trouble in winning them as well. 'It was an unbelievable experience for a barefoot boy, the son of a missionary, suddenly able to get virtually any girl he wanted,' he says. 'Many made written offers, like the letter I found recently in an old file: "I am 19 years old with blue eyes and was a Miss Brazil finalist last year. I know you are busy but I would like to meet you. Maybe one night you will call me and I come to your hotel for some time and some fun?" '[6]

As a boy, Barnard had once stood and stared at a wealthy man sitting next to a beautiful woman in the first-class cabin of a train standing in a station. He remembers dreaming of the day he would be like that. Thirty years on, his boyhood aspirations had become reality. He had been unfaithful to Louwtjie before the transplant but now Barnard became an unabashed playboy. On foreign trips, his high-level meetings were slotted around a seemingly endless series of sexual exploits with beauty queens, actresses and models. 'Just a few weeks previously I had only ever seen these beautiful Italian film stars in the movies,' he says. 'Now I was in and out of their bedrooms as if I'd been doing it all my life.'[7]

Barnard has written two autobiographies. The first, ghosted by Curtis Bill Pepper, is distinguished by its stylish writing. The second, by Barnard himself, is notable only for its bluntness. He reveals thoughts about women that, in today's non-sexist atmosphere, others might wish to bury, and uses language more in place in a steamy sex novel. He follows an air stewardess's 'undulating bottom' as she walks down the aisle in a plane. He recognizes a floor nurse by her 'firm slender body with urgent and inviting young breasts'. The actress Gina Lollobrigida, with whom he had a fling, runs her long nails down the front of his shirt and leans over him as he stares at the 'heaving swell of her breasts'. Jenny (no surname), an ex-Miss Italy, 'moaned softly as her tongue darted in and out of my mouth . . . Not even the cold weather could contain my excitement and she laughed wickedly . . . as she increased the pressure against my groin.'

In the end, it was all too much for Louwtjie. Possibly the final straw was her discovery of a love-letter from Gina Lollobrigida. The already strained marriage began to fall apart at the seams. 'I just decided I didn't want this any more,' she says. 'I didn't want all these women phoning me. I mean, when somebody phones you and says: "Look, sorry, he's not coming home tonight because he's spending the night with me." I thought: look, I must get rid of this guy . . . and while he was away I packed his things, phoned his office and when he came back I said: "No. I will name no woman. I just want a divorce and that's because I'll either land in an asylum or I'll take my own life and for my children's sake I can't do things like that. I don't want to do things like that. I just want to be Louwtjie.'

They divorced in 1969, after twenty-one years of marriage. Christiaan Barnard has twice remarried. He was seventy-three in November 1995 and now lives with Karin, his thirty-three-year-old wife, and their young son in a luxurious modern home equipped with a swimming pool on the outskirts of Cape Town. He also owns a farm. Barnard has few regrets about those turbulent years. 'Thinking back over the whole situation, if I had to do it over again, I don't think that I would change it very much,' he says. 'There is no doubt about it that being the surgeon who did the first heart transplant was worth every problem that I've had, because it's given me so much in life. I would not have what you see here today if it was not for the first transplant. It really made me what I am today. If I hadn't done it, I would have just been another heart surgeon in the world.'

Whatever people say about his personal life, Barnard will be remembered as the surgeon who had the courage and imagination to step into an area in which other surgeons were fearful of treading. In the weeks following the transplant at Groote Schuur Hospital, it was as if a dam had suddenly burst. Washkansky's new heart had been beating inside his chest for only two days when the second heart transplant took place. The man who did it was the man who had wanted to do the first: Adrian Kantrowitz.

'I kept thinking to myself,' Kantrowitz says, remembering the moment when he first heard the news of Barnard's operation, 'just because Chris has done a heart transplant is no reason for me not to do a heart transplant. It's perfectly reasonable. We've gotten all the permissions; we're all set; we have an appropriate donor; we have an appropriate recipient. So I decided in that half-hour to continue with our effort.'

Adrian Kantrowitz performed the world's second human heart transplant on 6 December 1967. Moral and legal qualms once again forced him to allow the donor child's heart to stop naturally before he opened its chest, but this time he decided to go ahead with the transplant: the heart looked all right. It took about forty-five minutes to give Jamie Scudero his new heart. It took another six and a half hours for the child to die after the operation.

'We were at the hospital in the waiting room,' says Jamie's mother, Anna, 'and then all of a sudden they were going crazy. Running here. Running there. And I said to my sister, "Oh, God, something must have happened." And that's when he came out and told me the baby's passed away. It was a tragedy . . . and you never get over it. Never get over it.'

Jamie's new heart had started and he had recovered from the anaesthetic, but the transplant was not strong enough to support his circulation. It had been too damaged, after all, says Kantrowitz, by being allowed to stop naturally. 'It would have made no difference to the donor if we had removed a beating heart . . . and it would have made a great deal of difference to the recipient,' he says. 'But that's the way the game was played in those days.'

Norman Shumway finally got his wish a month after Kantrowitz's operation. He found a private neurosurgeon willing to throw caution to the wind and sign the death certificate of a patient whose heart was beating but who had suffered irreversible brain damage. On 6 January 1968, Shumway became the third surgeon to transplant a human heart. But he did no better than the others. His patient, fifty-seven-year-old Mike Kasperak, survived just fifteen days before succumbing to internal bleeding.

Dark days lay ahead in transplant surgery – days in which cardiac surgeons in many countries jumped feet first onto the transplantation bandwagon. They had watched the transformation of Christiaan Barnard into the media's favourite doctor and they wanted a share of the action. The lure of fame proved a fatal attraction. Suddenly it seemed that you weren't a proper cardiac surgeon unless you were doing transplants. The operation became a status symbol. Moral and legal scruples about the removal of beating hearts were quickly forgotten in this medical gold rush. Nineteen sixty-eight was undoubtedly the year of the heart transplant: 102 operations were attempted by forty-seven different medical teams in eighteen countries as far apart as Venezuela, Australia and India. Even with undamaged hearts, the experience was a disaster. Forty of the patients transplanted in this period died within a week of their operations. Two-thirds were dead within three months. Only twenty-four lived longer than six months.[8] The surgeons who had paved the way for heart transplants by struggling for years to make the body accept a kidney looked on in horror.

'Everybody knows what a heart does,' says Francis Moore, who led the surgical department at the Peter Bent Brigham Hospital in Boston. 'Everybody knows where it is, and everybody realized that when it was transplanted, something terribly important had happened. Lots of people die of heart disease. So, two epidemics ensued. One was an epidemic that I call national chauvinism: every nation that did cardiac surgery wanted to show that they also could transplant the heart. And the other was an ego epidemic: some cardiac surgeons who knew absolutely nothing about transplantation, transplant immunity, antibody reactions or immuno-suppressive chemotherapy started to transplant the heart. There was an epidemic in this country that lasted about eighteen or twenty months . . . and that was a disaster.'

The difficulties of heart transplantation had been greatly underestimated. Because the surgery was relatively simple, many surgeons thought that once they had put a healthy heart in place, they should be able to manage rejection with drugs, much as the kidney transplanters were doing. However, kidney transplant patients could be placed back on dialysis (the artificial kidney) to keep them alive during a severe rejection crisis while there was no such temporary replacement for the heart. If it stopped for more than three or four minutes, the patient's brain was fatally damaged. In the early days, surgeons found the aftercare of their heart-transplant patients an unmanageable problem.

'It's only human nature that you want to be recognized and cheered and slapped on the back,' says Christiaan Barnard. 'And therefore they jumped in to do this operation with that idea in mind. Not so much for the patients but to be recognized, to be a celebrity. And unfortunately many did not know much about transplantation . . . I know of a unit that did a transplant and a doctor that worked there told me that, after a week, one of the doctors in that unit came to the head of department and said: "You know, I just read in the newspaper these patients should be treated for rejection." You see, they really didn't know what they were doing.'

Even where they did know about the delicate aftercare of transplant patients, it still went hopelessly wrong. British surgeons did not overcome their concern about entering the heart-transplant arena until May 1968, five months after Barnard's operation. They knew all about rejection, but the UK programme ran into difficulties from the start when Fred West was given the heart of a twenty-six-year-old carpenter. He did well for a month – so well that a euphoric transplant team waved 'I'm Backing Britain' flags at one of their press conferences. Then, shadows appeared in the X-rays of his lungs and the British doctors found themselves facing the same dilemma that Barnard had found impossible to resolve.

'We thought . . . it was something to do with rejection and we treated him more and more for rejection,' says Donald Long-more.[9] 'The reality of the situation was that he had clots forming in one of the chambers of his heart which were going off into his lungs. Now, when I look at those X-rays, it's so plain to see but . . . at that time we didn't have the sense to stop and say, "Now, just a minute, if this wasn't a transplant patient, if this was an ordinary chap, what would be going on here?" . . . It was understandable at the time, but tragic because had we anti-coagulated Fred instead of giving him massive immuno-suppressive drugs. I don't know, but he might have done better ... It gave the opposition to progress, to transplantation, an extra arrow to their bow – and it was a serious blow.'

A misdiagnosis contributed to Fred West's death forty-five days after his transplant and the British media turned on the surgeons they had once held in awe for attempting the impossible. The transplanters were condemned for doing too much too soon with too little knowledge about the consequences.

'Surely the time has come to call a halt to this procession of deaths,' wrote the *Times* medical correspondent the day after West's death. 'There can be no justification for an operation that carries such a devastatingly high mortality rate and the performance of which is more or less equivalent to a death sentence. . . . If the medical profession is not prepared to act itself then Parliament must step in.'[10]

'It is my opinion that in our present state of knowledge this operation should not be performed and it should never have been attempted,' carped Dr Abraham Marcus, then the *Observer*'s adviser on medical affairs.[11]

Dr Donald Gould, the editor of *New Scientist* magazine, condemned the 'dismal' results of heart-transplant surgery and called on the public to tell doctors they wanted a stop to 'these human experiments'. Malcolm Muggeridge, a writer, Christian and self-appointed guardian of moral standards in Britain, launched an uneducated but stinging attack on the very idea of removing a beating heart for transplantation. 'Once you start doing this, taking a heart from a virtually living person,' he said, 'it is a very slippery slope. Soon we shall be deciding: "This man is a loony. He has a good heart. His life is useless to him and we may as well have his heart." '[12]

The next two British heart-transplant patients fared little better. Gordon Forde was given his new heart in July 1968 and lived for only two days. Charles Hendrick managed to survive for five and a half months after his transplant in May 1969 – not long enough, though, to prevent the Department of Health from calling the British transplant programme to a halt until more progress had been made in fighting rejection. Another ten years passed before it started again.[13]

The man who performed the most heart transplants in this first heady year – and the man who received the most criticism – was Denton Cooley, a tall, imposing and highly skilled Texan doctor with a formidable reputation. He had already done several thousand open-heart operations at St Luke's Hospital in Houston, and never failed to amaze knowledgeable onlookers with his speed and precision. 'He's one of the giants in cardiovascular surgery,' says Jim Nora, a cardiologist who worked with Cooley at St Luke's in the 1960s. 'He has enormous energy and enormous confidence and enormous ability as a surgeon. . . . He's a very dedicated individual who is devoted to achieving innovation for as many patients as he can.' He also commanded great respect from his team. 'The staff, I think, were willing to do almost anything. If he said jump through a hoop, they were willing to do so,' says Dolly Guillot, one of the hospital's nurses. 'He really inspired everyone to do their best in whatever way that they were contributing, whether it be the housekeeping or preparing the foods in the kitchen and so forth. Everything was being done because Dr Cooley was the leader and in anything like this you have to have a leader.'

Cooley did not rush into the heart-transplant arena. His first took place in May 1968, when the world total already stood at eight. His first patient, Everett Thomas, recovered from the operation, went home a couple of weeks later, started work and lived for nearly seven months with the heart of a suicide victim beating inside his chest. 'He had moved to Houston for his recovery period,' remembers Cooley, 'and within about six weeks he was absolutely normal and in fact he got a job in one of our local banks and worked as a bank officer there for several months. I was most optimistic about it and was anxious to establish our position as one of the transplant centres in the world.'

Cooley put new hearts into seventeen patients in the last eight months of 1968, a sixth of the world's total that year. It was a peculiar combination of the character of the Texan surgeon and the pioneering spirit in Houston that sent St Luke's Hospital on this transplantation spree. 'Twenty-five years ago [Denton Cooley] didn't feel it was worth coming into the hospital unless he had at least ten patients to operate on,' says Jim Nora. 'He's just the sort of person who does a lot of work. He had the largest series of this, and the largest series of that. And so naturally he had the largest series of heart transplants initially. It was a time when we felt that anything was possible. We had the astronauts living in Houston and for some reason the heart transplanters were often thought of the same way, especially when invitations were given out. We might show up at the same parties even though we didn't know each other very well. . . . We were all very keyed up about what we were doing, thinking that it is important and may have infinite possibilities for the betterment of mankind.'

St Luke's Hospital began to act like a magnet on the country's cardiac patients. The motels and cheap hotels strung out on the main highways into Houston became temporary homes for the terminally ill, people who had heard of Cooley's transplants and had travelled to the city for the chance of life. Denton Cooley was their last hope. 'The hospital was bombarded with a lot of patients who were coming with their families from all parts of the United States,' says Guillot. 'They would listen for every ambulance that would come by and literally be hanging out waiting for the phone to ring telling them to come to the hospital, that there was a donor available for them. This was a last-ditch effort and they were willing to try anything that they could to prolong their lives and to live pretty much pain-free.'

It wasn't just the doctors and nurses who felt like pioneers. The publicity that each heart transplant attracted placed all the patients in the limelight. They, too, saw themselves as adventurers, explorers on a voyage into unknown territory. Few were shy about the media interest in their health and welfare. For most it was a blessed distraction from the daily struggle to survive. The problem was, most of these voyagers didn't return from their travels. Of the seventeen transplants Cooley did in 1968,[14] only three lived longer than six months. Nine died within a month of receiving their new hearts. Cooley's skill had been more than a match for the surgical challenge of heart transplantation – his lightning hands had reduced the average time of the operation from two hours to thirty minutes – but the immunological battle that faced the team in charge of the patient's after-care was an uphill struggle. They could not keep rejection at bay without opening their patients to overwhelming infection.

'Infections were a disastrous thing,' says Jim Nora. 'Herpes would just eat up some of these patients. The herpes virus would attack the face and then [they'd get] pneumonia from bacterial infection. What was successful in preventing rejection allowed the infection to come in. One patient who lived about five hundred days started out as a very muscular strong man, and there was so much of him to waste away. Instead of looking like a full-back, he appeared like someone who could have come out of Dachau.'

'Their bodies just rejected the hearts,' says Dolly Guillot. 'And the drugs weren't working. We were just really heartbroken because we weren't able to help them – and no amount of trying to console them seemed to work. Our hands were tied. We didn't know what to do. That was very difficult. I really wanted them to make it and when they died a part of me died as well.'

The transplant team continued in the face of these mounting disasters, hoping that the more information they gained from the operations, the more likely they would be to overcome the problems. Cooley's loyal troops followed their leader ever deeper into enemy territory, until the attrition rate became so high that dissension appeared in the ranks. Jim Nora stepped out of line and became one of the few voices arguing for a halt to the programme until they had found a better means of overcoming rejection. 'Denton realized too that we were having problems, but I guess he couldn't let go. We were all caught up in this idea that we can defeat death – and Denton was certainly leading the charge there. I think that he was looking for immortality. He was really not willing to accept that death was a possibility for any of his patients, for any of us, if you will. That's what we were trying to do, but we weren't successful. Death comes.'

The continuation of a medical programme that was producing so few benefits caused considerable conflict within St Luke's.

There was squabbling over what those on the outside of the transplant programme saw as a waste of precious hospital resources. Professional and personal relationships suffered in the inter-departmental bickering. 'Those who were not involved in transplants were rather indignant about the whole thing,' explains Jim Nora, 'and those who were involved in transplants were so busy, and maybe we were so filled with our own selves that we weren't aware of things that we should have been aware of. They'd say: "What are these people doing? Why all this craziness with transplant surgery? I mean, we've got all sorts of other surgery to do." People who used to be very congenial, saying, "Hello. How are you. It's good to see you", might avoid you in the hall. There was a fair amount of tension in that respect.'

Under pressure, Cooley eventually abandoned his programme in September 1969,[15] sixteen months after it had begun, and only when it became crystal clear that he was not going to solve the problem of rejection. He had given new hearts to twenty-one patients, only two of whom were still alive. It is clear now that it should have stopped much sooner than it did – even Cooley reluctantly admits that much. Looking back, he pins much of the blame for the failures on his poor choice of patients. Some of those given transplants were too ill to stand the trauma of the operation. Today Cooley would not offer such people a transplant. But why did he pursue the dream for so long in the face of such poor results? Cooley says, 'The real stimulus to continue were those few patients who felt absolutely marvellous and would go round extolling the virtues of cardiac transplantation. It's easy to criticize people who are inventors or discoverers, surgeons who are willing to take a chance. There's always professional jealousy involved and I admire people who will try new things and put their reputation on the line in order to achieve some purpose. . . . All of us in medicine are respectable and well-intentioned individuals [who] have a conscience about what we're doing . . . but at the same time we do have to utilize some of our opportunities to explore. And I believe, in an institution like this, that I have an obligation to remain on the cutting edge of progress.'

There are far less charitable views of Denton Cooley's sixteen-month, ill-fated adventure. Some kidney-transplant surgeons, who were watching these depressing developments with increasing anxiety, were outspoken in their criticism. 'I think it was a disgrace and I've said so in public,' Francis Moore says. 'They were superb operators but they didn't have any experience of transplant immunology. The Texans are good friends of mine – but they shouldn't have done all that so fast and I told them that at the time.'

At much the same time as the dissenting voices were growing in strength and number, a heart transplant took place in May 1968 at the Medical College of Virginia, in America, that placed the whole future of transplantation in doubt. A surgeon called Richard Lower[16] had tried to save the life of a young man dying of coronary artery disease with the healthy heart of a black man whose brain had been fatally damaged in an accident. It was, perhaps, inevitable that a doctor would, sooner or later, fall foul of the law. The ethical concerns that had prevented Adrian Kantrowitz and Norman Shumway from removing beating hearts from brain-dead bodies had been quickly forgotten after the first few heart transplants: the practical demands of the procedure, the need for undamaged hearts to give recipients the best chance of life, had won the argument in most hospitals. But in opening the chest of a patient who had previously been declared brain-dead and then removing their still beating heart, surgeons were skating on thin ice. They might have overcome their moral scruples, but they were turning a blind eye to the law of the land which, in 1968, still gave the heart a central role in the definition of death. Courts generally viewed this as 'a total stoppage of the circulation of the blood and a cessation of the animal and vital functions . . . such as respiration and pulsation'.[17]

It was Shumway's boy-scout definition – impractical, perhaps, in an age when high technology could keep hearts beating indefinitely inside hopelessly brain-damaged bodies – but the law nevertheless. So when Richard Lower removed Bruce Tucker's still beating heart on 25 May 1968, he was stepping into a legal minefield.

Tucker, a fifty-six-year-old labourer, had been drinking when he stumbled and fell in Richmond's Venable Street. His head hit a kerbstone and he was knocked unconscious. When he arrived at the Medical College of Virginia it was quickly apparent that his brain had been fatally damaged in the fall. Bruce Tucker's heart was beating, his blood pressure and temperature were normal. According to the traditional definition of death, he was very much alive – but the life in his body now depended on the ventilator that was forcing air in and out of his lungs. There was no electrical activity in his brain and, after a series of tests, neurologists in the hospital declared him brain-dead.

It was the opportunity for which Richard Lower had been waiting. He had been doing experimental heart transplants in dogs since 1960 and was looking for the chance to do his first clinical transplant. He had a patient, fifty-three-year-old Joseph Klett, whose only hope of survival was a transplant; now he had a potential donor.

'My colleagues and I spent the better part of two days trying to find – and have the police search for – members of the family because it was clear that he was brain-dead,' says Lower. 'We'd certainly hoped that when we did a transplant, everything would be perfect, including permission from the family. I think we tried very diligently and I don't know why they were not able to find the family.'

It is a mystery as to why the combined efforts of the Medical College of Virginia and the Richmond City Police Force were unable to locate a single relative. One of Bruce Tucker's sisters and two brothers lived in the city and it was stated in court that there was a business card inside his wallet containing the telephone number and address of one, William Tucker, who worked in a shoe shop just fifteen blocks from the hospital. However, in the absence of relatives, Virginia's chief medical examiner gave Richard Lower permission to remove Tucker's heart and transplant it into Joseph Klett. The examiner had checked the law books and found a local statute saying that unclaimed bodies could be used for medical purposes. It was the green light for Lower's first heart transplant – but when Bruce

Tucker's family discovered what had happened they saw red: they were only told that his heart had been removed when two of his brothers, Grover and William, went down to the undertaker's to retrieve his body.

'The boy running the funeral hall said: "Did you know the doctors have taken your brother's heart?"' says Grover Tucker. 'And, you know, that was a shocking thing. In other words, if it wasn't for the boy that worked at the funeral home, they'd have buried him and we'd have never known it. It was the worst thing that I could have thought could happen. You know, taking his heart without permission.'

The Tuckers found an outlet for their anger in a lawyer who'd also read the law books and discovered that, legally, death was still defined as the moment that the heart stopped. He agreed to sue Richard Lower and the transplant team for $100,000 for ending Bruce's life by removing his beating heart. It became a pivotal moment in the history of heart transplantation. If Lower lost, a legal precedent would be set that enhanced the boy-scout definition of death. The removal of beating hearts from brain-dead donors would become a much more risky undertaking. Heart-transplant surgeons would live in fear of the damage a court summons could do to their reputations and their bank balances, the exact problem that now faced Richard Lower.

'Well, it was a very serious case by the very nature of the allegations that the heart-transplant team had purposely killed Mr Tucker,' explains the trial judge, Justice A. Christian Compton. 'It was very serious – not only for Dr Lower but for the other physicians who were defendants in the case because at that time the transplantation of organs . . . certainly had not developed to the extent that it has today.'

The case was heard in 1972 in Richmond's Law and Equity Court before a jury of seven people, four years after Bruce Tucker's death. William Tucker's attorney outlined an emotional case to the jury. 'It was wrong to take Bruce Tucker's heart from his body,' he argued. 'They started the operation on Klett before Bruce Tucker was pronounced dead. They took the most precious thing he had going for him at the time, his heart.'[18]

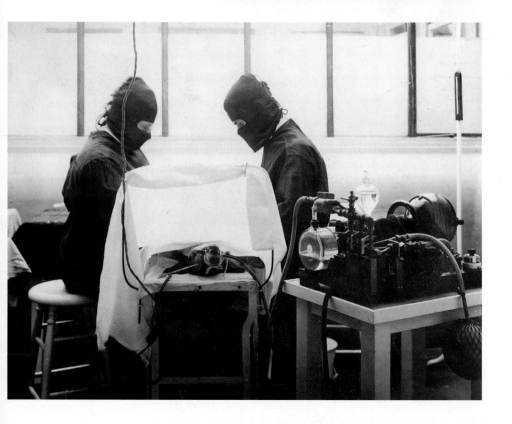

Right. Alexis Carrel: Nobel-prize-winning surgeon who did some of the earliest transplant experiments.

Below. Carrel with assistant operating on a dog in 1914.

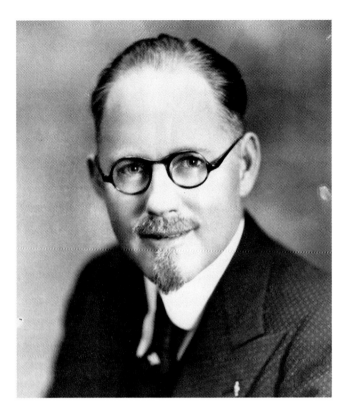

Left. John R. Brinkley: the 'quack' doctor who thought he could rejuvenate people by giving them testis transplants.

Below. Ruth Tucker (centre) on the day in July 1950 that she left hospital after her kidney transplant. Shown here with her husband and a nurse.

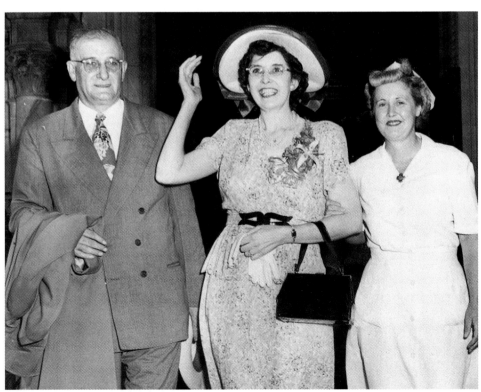

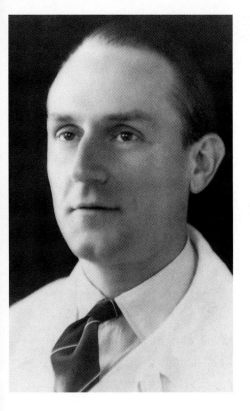

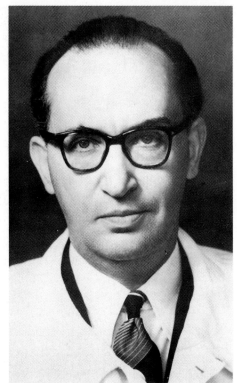

Above left. René Küss: the French surgeon who transplanted a kidney taken from a guillotined prisoner in 1951.

Above right. Jean Hamburger led the transplant team at the Necker Hospital in Paris in 1952. His first patient given a new kidney lived for just twenty-one days.

Right. David Hume: gave new kidneys to nine patients in Boston between 1951 and 1953. All died early deaths except one who lived for almost six months.

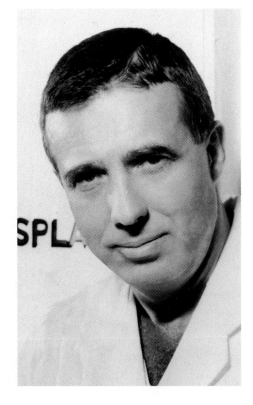

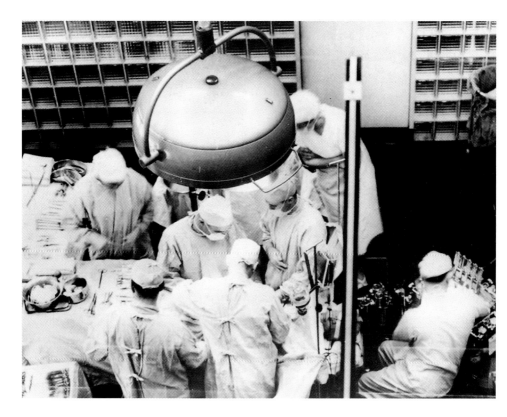

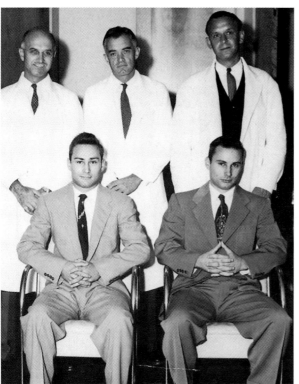

Above. Joseph Murray operating on Richard Herrick in Boston in 1954.

Left. Richard Herrick (front row, left) seen here with the donor of his transplanted kidney, his identical twin Ronald and (back row, left) Joseph Murray, the surgeon who gave it to him. They are pictured with two other members of the transplant team that did the world's first successful kidney transplant in 1954.

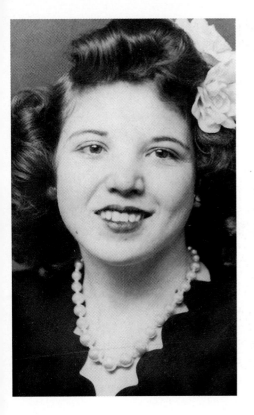

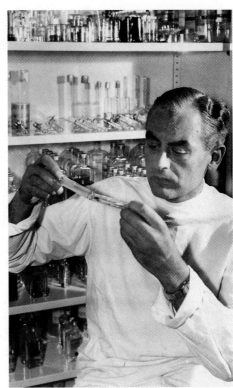

Above left. Gladys Lowman: the first patient to be given X-rays to prevent rejection. She died twenty-eight days after her transplant in 1958.

Above right. Peter Medawar. The zoologist who first showed that rejection could be beaten. He was knighted in 1960.

Right. Roy Calne: the surgeon who helped find the first practical method of preventing rejection in patients. Shown here in 1960 with Lollipop, one of this longest-surviving kidney transplant dogs.

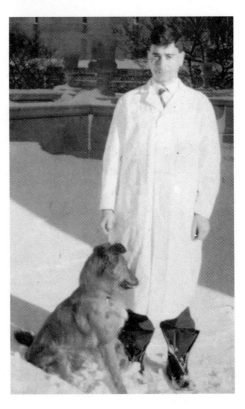

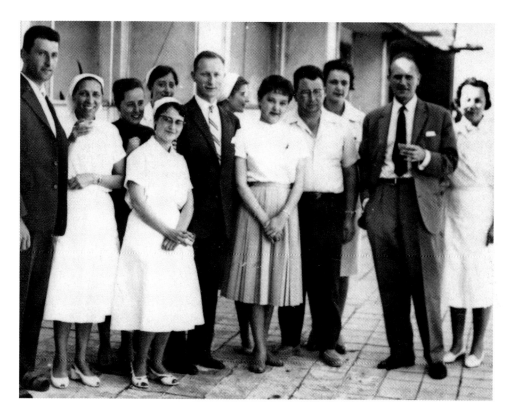

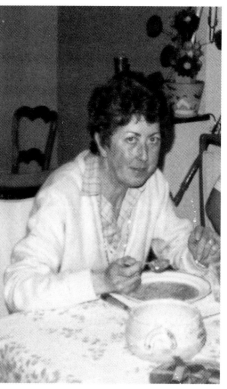

Above. Mrs Gen (centre) with René Küss (second from right). She was the first person to live for more than a year on a kidney transplanted from a completely unrelated donor.

Left. Yvette Thibault: she's lived longer than anyone else in the world with a kidney transplanted from an unrelated donor. Her operation was in October 1964.

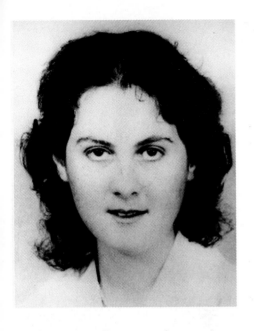

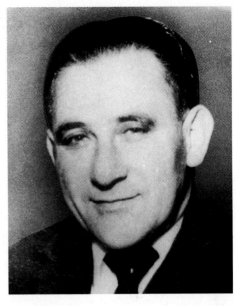

Denise Darvall: run over by a car in Cape Town in December 1967. She was the donor in the world's first human heart transplant.

Louis Washkansky: given Denise Darvall's heart in 1967 in an operation that changed the face of transplant surgery.

The team that did the world's first human heart transplant in December 1967. Chris Barnard is standing fourth from right in the middle row.

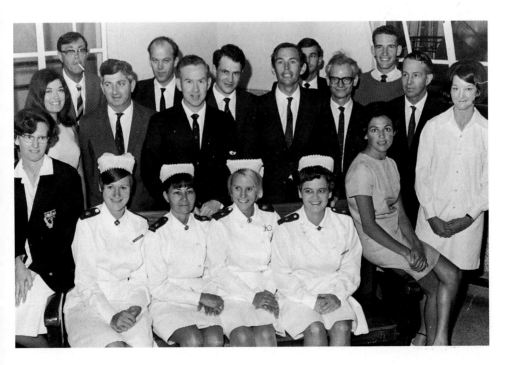

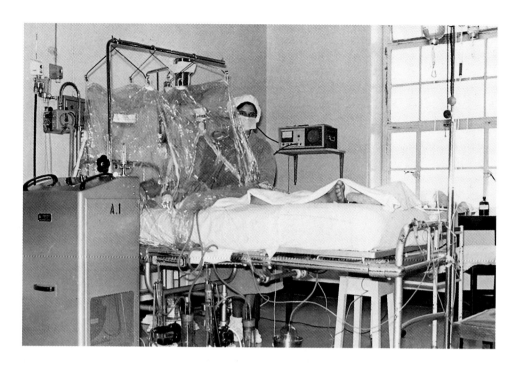

Louis Washkansky under an oxygen tent shortly after his transplant operation in December 1967.

Jamie Scudero, the second person to be given a new human heart. He died six and a half hours after his transplant at Maimonides Medical Centre in New York.

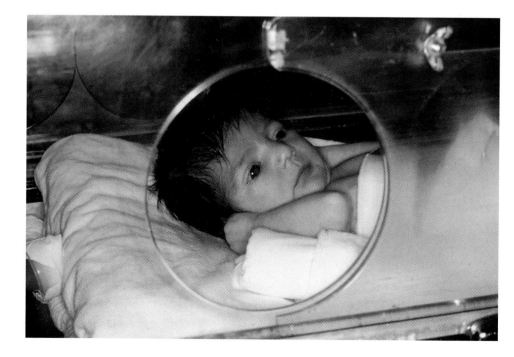

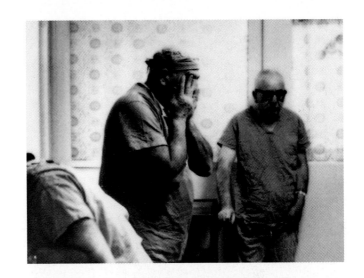

Adrian Kantrowitz (centre) after his first heart transplant on Jamie Scudero in December 1967. The operation was a failure.

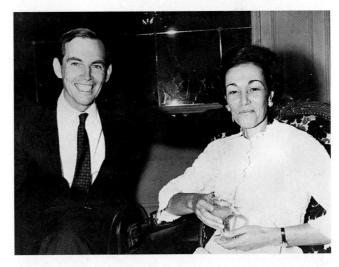

Chris and Louwtjie Barnard – in happier days before their separation.

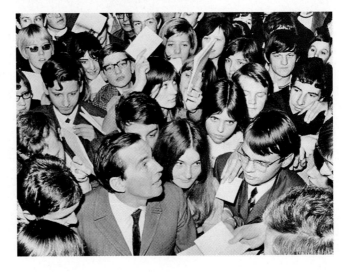

Chris Barnard besieged by young autograph hunters in Germany in 1968.

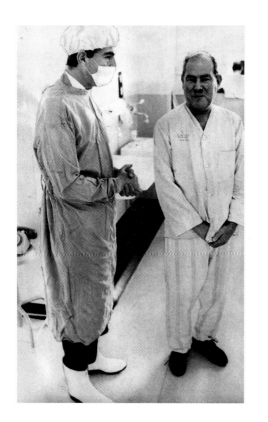

Left. The first picture of Philip Blaiberg after his heart transplant in January 1968. He's shown here with Chris Barnard.

Below. Showing the flag for Britain. The transplant team at the National Heart Hospital in London at a press conference after the first British heart transplant in May 1968.

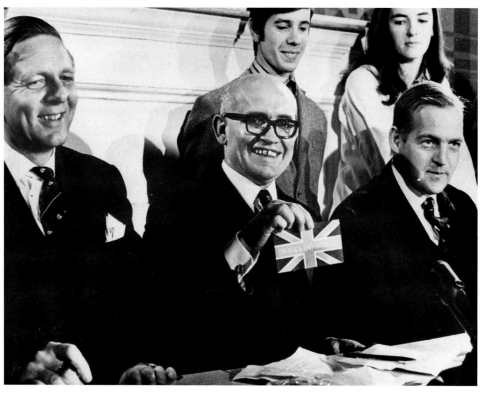

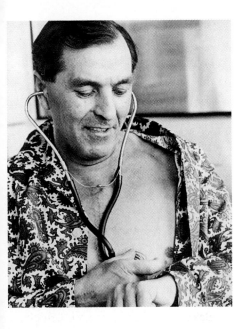

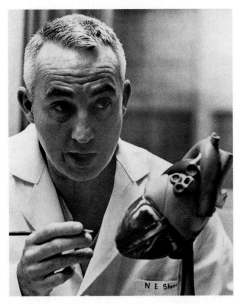

Fred West, Britain's first heart transplant patient. He lived just forty-five days after his operation in May 1968.

Norman Shumway, the heart surgeon from California who carried on transplanting hearts when almost everyone else had stopped.

Everett Thomas, Denton Cooley's first heart transplant patient, shortly after his operation in 1968.

Denton Cooley: he did more heart transplants in the last eight months of 1968 than anyone else in the world. Most of his patients died early deaths.

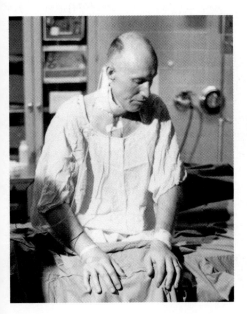

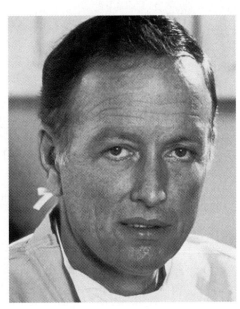

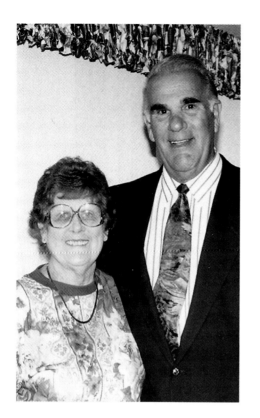

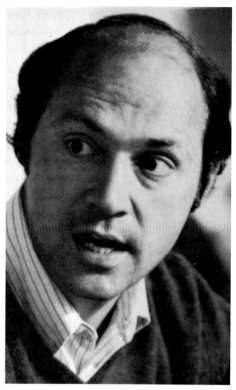

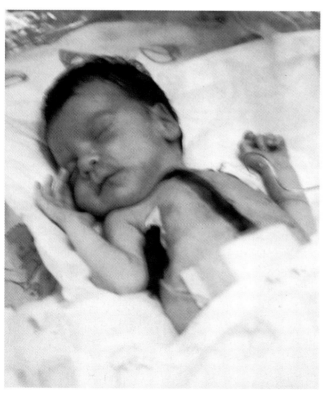

Above left. Lorraine Ustipak with John Najarian, the surgeon who bucked the system to save her life. Photographed in 1994.

Above right. William Summerlin – the researcher who was sacked for faking his results.

Left. Baby Fae: a baboon's heart couldn't save her life.

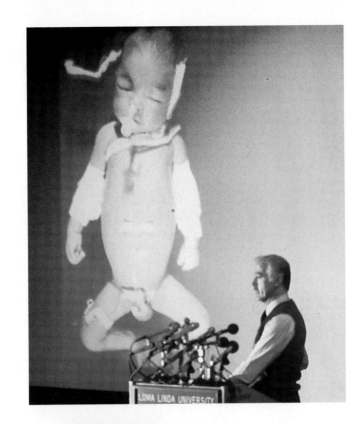

Leonard Bailey – life threatened after transplanting a baboon's heart into a baby girl.

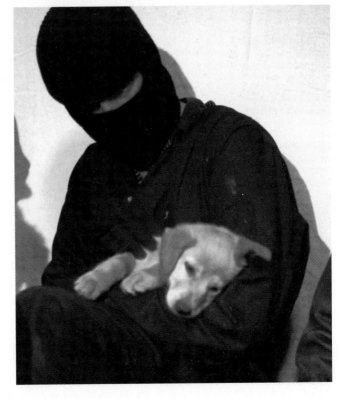

A member of the militant Animal Liberation Front shown here after raiding Leonard Bailey's laboratory at Loma Linda University to free experimental animals.

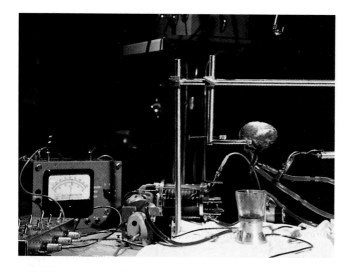

A monkey's brain removed from its skull and mechanically kept alive outside the body by the American neurosurgeon Robert White.

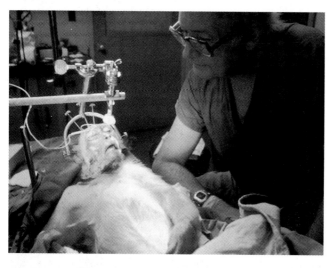

Robert White, pictured here with the body of one monkey that has been transplanted on to the head of another.

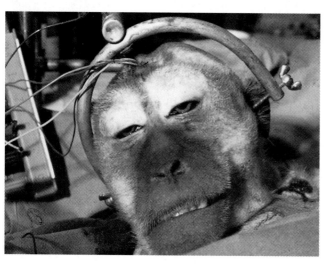

Another of White's whole body transplants. This one regained consciousness.

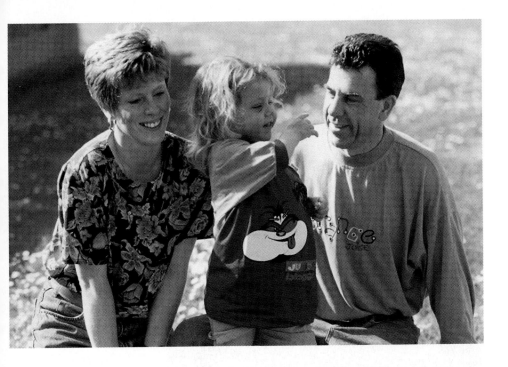

Laura Davies – the little English girl who died after surgeons in Pittsburgh, USA, transplanted six organs into her body. Shown here with her mother and father.

Benito Agrelo: the boy who decided to die rather than suffer the side effects of his anti-rejection drugs.

Betty Baird (left) – the liver transplant patient who threw away all her anti-rejection drugs and lived.

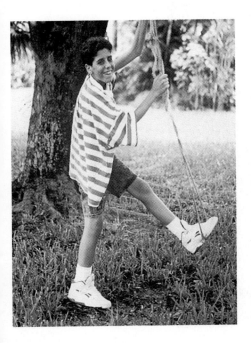

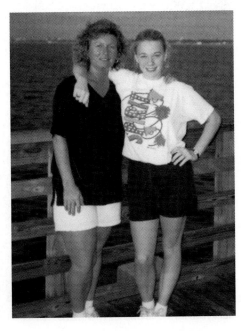

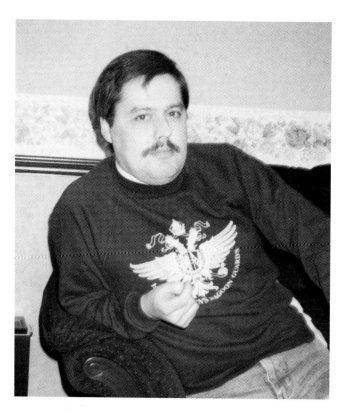

Left. Stephen Hyett: the man whose life was saved by six transplanted organs.

Below. Imutran's genetically engineered pigs. Soon, their organs could be saving people's lives.

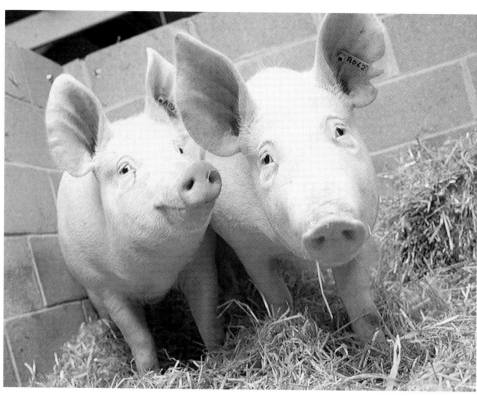

The core issue was the question of brain-death, and whether the jury would be allowed to consider this in determining the moment of Bruce Tucker's demise. The judge faced a serious dilemma: the legal definition of death – the cessation of heartbeat – was unambiguous. The law did not recognize any such concept as brain-death. Why should he let the jury use it in their deliberations? Judge Compton made up his mind after hearing some of the expert witnesses called by the transplant team to support their case. 'The evidence was clear, from their standpoint,' he says, 'that the medical profession at that time, in 1972, recognized as one of the criteria for the time of death, whether or not there was an irreversible loss of brain function. And so I felt that it was vital that the jury decide whether they would accept the traditional criteria, excluding brain-death, or whether, under the evidence in the case, brain-death should be included as part of the definition.'

Judge Compton had decided effectively that current medical practice in the determination of death was a more important principle to uphold than a dictionary definition. The jury was instructed to consider brain-death alongside the traditional view in determining the moment that Bruce Tucker lost his life. After an hour's discussion, they decided that Bruce Tucker had already died at the time his heart was removed. His family left the courtroom with serious misgivings about the good intentions of some of America's leading transplant surgeons. 'There's nothing they can say to make me believe they didn't kill him,' Bruce's brother, William, complained after the hearing.[19]

But Richard Lower and the rest of America's heart-transplant community, breathed a heavy sigh of relief.

'I think it was important,' says Lower, 'because there had been no court test of the legal definition of death. Had the court decided for some reason that we had to stick to the original definition, then I think virtually every surgeon would have been reluctant to remove a beating heart for a transplant. Patients would have died[20] and progress would have stopped.'

The verdict in Lower's case formalized the revolution that was taking place in America and elsewhere in our understanding of the moment of death. It was also a milestone in the development of heart transplantation. Within months, the state of Virginia – where the trial took place – had introduced legislation that made brain-death an acceptable medical concept. Other US states followed suit. 'It certainly put an end to a successful attack on surgeons engaged in heart transplantation on the ground that was alleged in this case – that is, that they in effect killed the donor in order to get his heart,' says Judge Compton.

By the end of the 1960s, many other countries were also using brain-death to determine the ending of life. Japan was a notable exception. Three months after Lower's ill-fated transplant, the medical world there had been engulfed in a second legal scuffle over brain-death. It was a similar story: a surgeon taken to task for removing the beating heart of a man who had suffered irreversible brain damage. But the Japanese people's unique feelings about life and death ensured a very different outcome for the nation's fledgling transplant community. To this day, the new heart that Professor Juro Wada gave to eighteen-year-old Miyazaki Nobuo on 8 August 1968 remains Japan's first and only heart transplant.

The patient recovered sufficiently to enjoy wheelchair-bound strolls in the hospital grounds but he died of a lung infection around three months later. It was after his death that Professor Wada's problems arose. The donor of Miyazaki's heart had been a twenty-one-year-old who had failed to regain consciousness after a swimming accident. A physician at Sapporo Medical College, where the transplant took place, raised serious questions about the Professor's treatment of the donor. He criticized Wada for not trying hard enough to save the swimmer's life and for cutting open the donor's chest before receiving the family's consent to remove the heart. The claims struck a chord in Japan, where differing religious beliefs had combined to create a strong aversion to transplantation. In the Shinto tradition, for example, bodies are supposed to be buried or cremated intact. Confucianism says that living family members should bear responsibility for any harm that comes to their dead relatives' remains. And Buddhism teaches that the corpse remains the dwelling place of a

person's mind and soul until a certain period of time has elapsed
after the heart has stopped. Hence bodies must be buried intact.
Many Japanese even object to the idea of an autopsy to discover
the cause of death and see organ transplantation as little more
than the desecration of the body of a loved one. It was hardly
surprising that a few weeks after the death of Japan's first heart
transplant patient, a law-suit had been filed against Wada
charging him with murder.

The case never came to trial as there wasn't enough evidence
to prove that the donor would have survived had his heart not
been removed. Wada was let off the hook – but transplant
surgery was strangled at birth in Japan, killed by a mixture of
religious tradition and an ever-present threat of prosecution.
Before they dropped the case, the local public prosecutor's office
threw out the idea of brain-death. They ruled instead that
terminal heart failure was the only way to define the end of life.
In the past quarter-century, hardly any surgeon has been willing
to risk their freedom and their career by removing an organ
from beating-heart cadavers. The few who have, have all faced
criminal investigations.[21] The only organ that may be transplanted in Japan is the kidney, because it can be taken from the
body after the heart has stopped beating or given as a gift by a
live donor.[22]

Despite the controversies and repeated failures, the hopes of
the world's transplant teams were kept alive by isolated triumphs,
people who had been brought back from the brink of death and
whose lives were genuinely transformed by their new hearts. The
handful of victories made dramatic headlines and helped to dispel
some of the disappointment of defeat. Perhaps the most famous
long-term survivor was Philip Blaiberg, the fifty-eight-year-old
South African dentist who became Christiaan Barnard's second –
and the world's third – heart-transplant patient on 2 January
1968. In the weeks leading up to his operation, he was very sick. 'I
went to see him one day in the hospital,' remembers his sister-in-
law, Anne Gordon. 'He was gasping for breath. He was under an
oxygen tent all the time. He had no chance of ever living, you
know, except day to day . . . If something serious had not been

done to him, he would never have lived longer than a week or so. The transplant came just in the nick of time, I think.'

Blaiberg was given the heart of Clive Haupt, a twenty-five-year-old coloured man who had suffered a fatal brain haemorrhage. The transplant team had overcome their fear of using a non-white person's heart for their second transplant, but there was a subtle irony in the use of a coloured donor. Under South Africa's racist apartheid laws, Groote Schuur Hospital was segregated: whites went in at a different entrance and were treated in a different part of the hospital from blacks and coloureds. In life, Haupt's body was not allowed to cross the racial divide, but no law prevented his heart from giving new life to a sick white man. Only in death, therefore, could the body of this coloured man be brought into the whites only part of the hospital, to lie in an operating theatre next door to Philip Blaiberg in preparation for the transplant.

Blaiberg was the first heart-transplant patient to recover from his operation and be allowed home.[23] He left Groote Schuur Hospital on 16 March, ten weeks after receiving his new heart. By then, five other human-heart transplants had been attempted, but the patients had died in hospital within hours or days of their operations. Blaiberg's trip home to his apartment in Wynberg, Cape Town, was a major media event.

'I had been told the world press and television teams were waiting outside with hundreds of citizens who had gathered hours before to give me a rousing welcome and send-off,' Blaiberg recalled. 'I had no intention of allowing the world to see Professor Barnard's patient leave the hospital in a wheelchair. No. I would use my legs. I raised myself out of the chair and walked steadily towards the door and outside. I felt elated and a new vigour seemed to flow through me as I passed over the threshold into the world I had yearned for so long.'[24]

Philip Blaiberg became a tourist attraction in Cape Town. The rich and famous beat a path to his door to shake hands with the living proof that new hearts could indeed be swapped for old. His phone rang endlessly with calls from the local and international press. He went swimming and kicked a rugby ball around for the TV cameras. The man who had once been so sick he could barely catch his breath, now had the hopes of the transplant world resting on his shoulders.

'Well, he almost became a young man,' says Anne Gordon. 'He went for walks a long way along the beach and, you know, walking on sand is not easy. He managed all that. He went for drives. Apparently he took Chris Barnard for a drive one day. He was game for everything. He was bright, he was social, he went out, he missed nothing. He had a wonderful year which he never would have had.'

However, the anti-rejection drugs that Blaiberg was taking could only slow the progress of the inevitable, not prevent it. As his new heart gradually became less efficient, his good health and renewed vigour disappeared. Blaiberg died from chronic rejection in August 1969, eighteen months after his operation. But his long survival had lit a beacon of hope for the transplant community.

'I think that if we had failed with that operation, we would have put transplantation back a long way,' commented Christiaan Barnard. 'We had to show that a patient who underwent a cardiac transplant was able to recover from the operation, was able to leave hospital, to lead a normal life. And, with the luck that we had, that is what we managed to show in Dr Blaiberg. . . . He was the first patient to live a year after transplantation. And this encouraged surgeons in other parts of the world to take up this operation in great seriousness. If we'd failed . . . I think I would have had so much pressure from the rest of the hospital and medical staff that I would have had to stop.'

Barnard performed few heart transplants in these early years: he gave just six patients new hearts between December 1967 and May 1971. But his results outshone everyone else's. Four of the six lived for more than a year after their operations. Dorothy Fisher was transplanted on 17 April 1969 and survived for twelve years. Dirk Van Zyl received his new heart on 10 May 1971 and lived for twenty-three years. Careful selection of patients and meticulous after-care contributed to these good results. With many other surgeons finding it hard to keep their patients alive for more than a month or two, Barnard should have been seen as a source of valuable experience and advice, but his new-found fame and the gossipy newspaper accounts of his personal life reflected badly on his reputation. He says he felt completely ostracized, particularly by the Americans. 'There were units who were actually very much against what we did and to some extent were very jealous,' he says. 'There was this feeling, especially in the United States, that one of the surgeons there should have been the first to do a transplant . . . I don't understand that because we were as well prepared as they were. But they were openly against us.'

Despite these few successes, by 1969 a cold realism had replaced the over-enthusiasm and media hype that had greeted the first heart transplants. It was now glaringly obvious that the body of wisdom gained from the care of kidney-transplant patients was not sufficient to make heart transplantation an accepted therapy. The balancing act was exceptionally delicate: it could be made to work, but the path between rejection and infection was narrow and the casualties far too high. In the second full year of heart-transplant surgery, the number of operations more than halved: only forty-seven were done in 1969; thirty-four of the patients died within three months of their operations; only eight lived longer than six months. By 1970, transplant surgery's affair of the heart had almost ground to a halt. World-wide, just sixteen heart transplants took place in the first ten months of the year: only five survived for more than six months.[25] By the end of the year, few of the sixty-five different surgical teams were left in the game. One that did not quit was the team at Stanford University Medical Centre led by Norman Shumway, whose extensive experimental work had paved the way for Barnard's pioneering operation on Louis Washkansky. Shumway had come under considerable pressure to abandon the work but continued doggedly to pursue his dream of making heart transplantation a life-saving operation. The American College of Cardiology wanted a moratorium on heart transplants and even the president of the board of trustees of his own university wanted him to stop. But Shumway won through, and, where so many other cardiac surgeons gave up in despair, he worked slowly and methodically to overcome the problems. 'We didn't stop because the patients were living,' he says. 'We didn't do two or three transplants a week. We'd do one and then we'd work very carefully with that patient. Then a month later we'd do the next one. That was the way to do it. We had the experimental background and we knew this thing would work.'

Even during the disastrous first two years, Shumway's results were well above average: four of the five long-term heart transplant survivors in 1970 were transplanted at Stanford. Progress was unspectacular but consistent. The experience gained from each operation made it a little easier to walk the fine line between rejection and infection. Each year the statistics improved. In 1968 22 per cent of Shumway's heart-transplant patients survived for more than a year. By 1976, 71 per cent of his patients – nearly two-thirds – were still alive twelve months after their transplants. A third were surviving five years or more.[26] Heart transplantation was emerging from the dark ages and even the most sceptical of critics began to recognize its worth as a life-saving therapy.

But by the middle of the 1970s the kidney was still the only organ routinely being transplanted. The heart and the liver were still considered experimental and the handful of attempts to transplant organs like the pancreas, the intestines and the lungs had failed. Surgeons had to wait for a revolution in the after-care of their patients before transplantation could move out of second gear.

5

The Holy Grail

The side effects of the drugs that kept transplant patients alive were a source of endless worry to the doctors charged with keeping rejection at bay. The two most widely used in 1970 were Imuran,[1] which kills the cells responsible for destroying a transplanted organ, and Prednisone,[2] a steroid that can disrupt a variety of immune responses. Steroids were particularly useful in helping a patient overcome a rejection crisis when Imuran failed to prevent their body from mounting an intense attack against the transplant. High doses of Prednisone would often damp down the immune response and help the patient survive the onslaught. Some people, however, required large amounts of the drug administered over long periods and there was frequently a high price to pay for their survival.

Betty Baird knows about the cost. She had suffered from chronic hepatitis, a disease she had caught in childhood and which had progressively damaged her liver to the point where her options had narrowed to a transplant or death. The new liver Betty received in Denver, Colorado, when she was twenty saved her, but the anti-rejection drugs made her life a misery. The steroids were the culprits: her face swelled, she ate continuously, put on a lot of weight and became very self-conscious about her appearance. Most upsetting for her and her family was the character change that the drugs caused. 'They affected me real bad,' she says. 'My mother was the one who pointed out my mood changes – one minute I would be laughing hysterically and the next I would be screaming. I got divorced as my husband could not handle me being sick,' Betty explains, from her home in Union Town, Pittsburgh.

Her mother, Jane Bradey, remembers the disturbing transformation of her daughter: 'You would have to watch Betty real closely as the slightest thing would make her cry,' she says. 'She had real bad ups and downs. If I paid more attention to one of her daughters she would say to me, "You don't love me", that sort of thing. She was not like that before. Betty was always very cheerful and an outgoing person and this was such a drastic change.'

Betty Baird's problems were far from unique. 'In most centres that you go to they will say: "Our side effects? Well, we manage them pretty well," ' says David White, an immunologist at Cambridge University. 'But the side effects from those huge doses of steroids could be appalling. Cushing's syndrome: almost every single patient had round faces and big bloated bodies. You get diabetes. You get psychoses. You get gastric ulcers. You get sterile bone necrosis – the bones crumble. You don't get all of these in every patient, but these are the side effects. Of course, tremendous risks from infection. Poor wound healing. Just a gamut of symptoms.'

The side effects of Imuran, while not quite as bad, could be serious enough. Used in too high a dose, it could damage the liver or bone-marrow. Used at levels the body could tolerate, it was sometimes unable to keep rejection at bay. Then, to save their patients' lives, doctors had little choice but to reach for the toxic steroids. Rejection had been placed in a chemical strait-jacket – but it always threatened to break out and, ultimately, the effort to keep it caged made prisoners of the transplant patients themselves. It was an uneasy balance.

A new approach was needed and by 1970 medical researchers in several different countries were exploring ways of muting the body's immune system without making victims of the patients. It amounted to a quest for immunology's Holy Grail: a means of preventing rejection that has no unwanted side effects. Such a discovery would transform the lives of thousands of people and, of course, bring recognition to the man or woman who found the key.

One approach was tissue typing, the attempt to match the tissues of donor and recipient, much as blood groups are matched before giving a transfusion. The closer the match, the less likely was the body to react strongly against the transplant. That, at least, was the theory that had been worked out by Jean Dausset, a French scientist who won the Nobel Prize in 1980 for his efforts.[3] It had already been shown to work in mice[4] and in 1970 most immunologists believed that if surgeons only transplanted well-matched organs, their patients' chances of survival would increase dramatically. It seemed a sensible theory, and many kidney-transplant surgeons began to tissue type their patients and refuse to use organs that were poor matches. But there was always a shortage of transplantable organs and some surgeons felt it was a crime to make seriously ill patients wait even longer than they already had to for a well-matched organ. Dr John Najarian, a transplant surgeon working at the University of Minnesota Medical School in Minneapolis, believed that the most important factor in a successful transplant was the condition of the organ. If it appeared healthy, he was prepared to offer it to a patient whatever the tissue match – and whatever the tissue typers might say. 'The rest of the medical profession kind of looked down upon us for doing these transplants,' says Najarian. '[They] felt that we weren't going to succeed with these poor matches.'

Najarian didn't listen to the tissue typers, because he had been checking the tissue matches of the organs that he put into his transplanted patients to see who did well and who did not. The results in his clinic cast considerable doubt on the theory of tissue matching. Some patients who by chance had been given well-matched organs died rapidly after their operations; others with poorly matched organs survived for many years. Lorraine Ustipak is one of them. She developed an incurable kidney disease in the late 1960s and was told that she didn't have long to live. In those days, the artificial kidney was still in its infancy and could be used only for a short period without causing serious complications. A transplant was her only hope and she began the nail-biting wait for a suitable donor. Her near relatives couldn't help: some would not risk sacrificing a kidney and those who were happy to do so had incompatible blood groups. Lorraine Ustipak thought she would have to wait for someone to die before getting her trans-plant – until a distant cousin offered to save her life. 'I was in bed I remember, at the time, in my room and [my husband] called me and told me that Vivian wanted to give me her kidney. Unbelievable! I've thought about it many times and every time I talk about it I have this emotional outburst. But it's just unavoidable. I can't help it. Even many years afterwards.'

In 1969, Najarian's team transplanted one of Vivian's kidneys into Lorraine's body. In doing so they trod heavily on the tissue typers' toes. 'Her cousin was not a good tissue match,' says Najarian. 'As a matter of fact there were no similarities whatsoever but we felt we should proceed with that transplant, that it would be better than anything we could get from someone who had recently died, [from] a cadaver. Well, today, here we are, twenty-six years later, Lorraine Ustipak is doing beautifully. She has a normally functioning kidney and other than taking one or two pills a day is a normal individual. Had we listened to the tissue typers . . . I think she would have died on dialysis and she wouldn't be with us today. Since that time we have had many others like Lorraine Ustipak who have no match and who have a perfect kidney.'

Tissue typing only worked, Najarian believed, if there was a perfect match between the tissues of donor and recipient.[5] Patients transplanted in these circumstances were then much more likely to survive. But perfect matches were exceptionally rare[6] and, in his experience, there was no correlation between survival time and anything less than perfect matching.[7] 'From a practical point of view, in our own programme here, where everything is exactly the same, [where] the operations are done by the same surgeon, for example, so that there is no bias, we have found that it doesn't make any difference what the match is,' Najarian explains. 'The poorly matched kidneys did just as well as the well-matched kidneys, that is, with the exception of the . . . perfect match . . . I think that the best thing to look for is a good kidney in a good institution – this is better than anything else you can do. By a good kidney, I mean a kidney that is not injured in its period of removal. Finding a good physiological organ is the best thing you can do.'

In 1970 such comments amounted to heresy. The theorists were adamant that matching the tissues of donor and recipient was possibly the most hopeful way of sparing patients from the debilitating effects of high doses of chemical immuno-suppression. It was, therefore, relatively easy to dismiss the views of one surgeon. When Paul Terasaki, one of the leaders in the field of tissue typing, stood up and publicly backed Najarian's clinical findings, though, the world of immunology was thrown into uproar. Within months of taking his stand, the heavy hand of officialdom tried to throw Terasaki out of business. It was only with great ingenuity that he kept open his laboratory at the University College of Los Angeles.

Since the mid 1960s, Paul Terasaki and his colleagues had been identifying human tissue types and using them to try to predict the success of a transplant. The theory was clear: the closer the tissue match, the better the patient's chances of survival. It was a sliding scale of success: from perfect A matches with the best chance of a successful transplant down to poorly matched F transplants, which should have the least. The problem was that Terasaki, like Najarian, was unable to make the theory work. For six years he had been receiving tissue samples from donors and recipients of livers transplanted by Tom Starzl at the Veterans' Administration Hospital in Denver, Colorado. He had built up a database of a thousand different tissue types, but all he could say with certainty was that, apart from close blood relatives, patients whose kidneys came from *perfectly* matched donors needed less immuno-suppression and survived longer than those whose organs did not. Other than that, he couldn't predict anything. There was no sliding scale of success. Patients with *poorly* matched kidneys were as likely to do well as those with *reasonably* matched ones.

'When we first started to do tissue typing, of course we expected it to work,' he says. 'And one of the things that was surprising was about half the patients that we knew were definitely mismatched seemed to have good results. We were hesitant to report this but finally by 1970 we had so many examples of this that we felt we had to . . . speak up about it.'

There was some urgency to this decision. In Italy, the supporters of tissue typing were trying to get a law passed to make it illegal to transplant an organ without first matching the tissues of donor and recipient, which would pave the way for similar legislation in many other countries – legislation that Terasaki believed would deny patients the organs that might save their lives. His opportunity came at a conference in The Hague in September 1970, six years after he started trying to unravel the tissue-typing system in humans.

'I felt I had no choice [but] to say what we found even though everybody else was very upset and angry about it,' says Terasaki. 'I think the tendency was for everybody to assume we weren't doing the tests right. They thought, this is the basic theory and if you get it right you should get the right answer. That's what everybody felt. Actually we had spent a lot of time trying to ensure that we were doing it correctly, that this wasn't an artefact of the laboratory. A lot of people in the tissue-typing community were upset.'

That was no surprise. One of the top tissue typers, a man who had staked his reputation on a belief in the value of tissue typing, was now saying that the system didn't work. Not that it couldn't work, only that the system wasn't sufficiently understood at present to make it work. But that didn't alter the grim reception that most delegates gave Terasaki's speech.

'I suspect that if anyone had had tomatoes they would have pitched them at him,' says Tom Starzl, who was at the meeting, 'because for the most part the audience consisted of people who had built in the idea that matching was going to be an effective discriminating instrument of organ allocation . . . I suppose my primary emotion when I heard him speak in The Hague was love or affection for somebody who had the courage to essentially commit professional suicide in order to tell the truth about a matter in which the consensus was all in another direction.'

The speech ignited a fierce controversy. The chair of the conference, Jon Van Rood, another leading tissue typer from Holland, told Terasaki point blank that he had drawn the wrong conclusions from incomplete data. 'I told him that it was unwise to present the data in this way because of the many uncertainties,' explains Van Rood. 'The research was done with few patients and, at the time, we didn't know how to analyse the data correctly. So he should have been careful not to give the information in such a way that people jumped to hard conclusions. And their conclusion was that tissue matching did not matter . . . even though there are many facts which argue against this . . . I felt that the picture was not as black and white as he presented it.'

The tissue typers may have been incensed but many surgeons took a different view. One came up to Van Rood after the meeting, described Terasaki's speech as a 'bloody good talk' and said how marvellous it was that he didn't have to worry about that 'damn matching any more'. It was a common view. Surgeons faced with dying patients did not want to be prevented from using viable organs. And, anyway, they thought that tissue typing patients waiting for new hearts and livers was not practical as there was no means of keeping them alive for long periods while they waited for a suitable match.

'We surgeons were very positive about Terasaki's presentation,' says John Najarian, 'because we were then, as we are to this day, faced with a severe donor-organ shortage. Tissue typers wanted to wait for perfect matches, for the best match. We like to use every organ as we feel that poorly matched do as well as well-matched. Terasaki showed in his presentation . . . very strong evidence for what we had already found. It meant that we could use every organ that we had. Of course [it] was considered heresy among the tissue typers. If your only tool is a hammer and someone tells you that hammers are not necessary, then of course you will react hostilely.'

Two days after the conference ended in The Hague, Tom Starzl flew back to America, stopping off briefly at London's Heathrow airport. He was doing some duty-free shopping there when he recognized an official of the National Institutes of Health, the body funding Terasaki's work. The official, also returning from the conference, was deep in conversation with another man in the airport book-shop and did not notice Starzl. When Terasaki's name cropped up in the conversation, Tom Starzl's ears pricked up. 'What I heard fixed that moment in my brain to the smallest detail,' says Starzl. 'The two were planning an emergency site visit to UCLA with the intention of discontinuing Terasaki's laboratory support. Paul's heretical report was not what they wanted to hear, and now the messenger must be killed.'[8]

Starzl phoned Terasaki to warn him of the plan and, sure enough, several weeks after the meeting at The Hague, twenty NIH officials descended on his laboratory. There was little he could do to change the course of events. On Christmas Eve 1970 Terasaki's $400,000 grant was abruptly withdrawn. As the NIH was his only source of income, the country's leading tissue typer was being fired for telling what he believed to be the truth. 'This was a scientific piece of work,' says Terasaki, 'and I felt I had to say what actually existed but I didn't think that the funds that I was receiving from the NIH would be affected by this. . . . Some people in the Government perhaps thought that, as we hadn't come out with the answers they expected, we should not continue to be funded. . . . Since that time we have not received funds for this kind of work.'

Terasaki believed that, given time and resources, he could make tissue typing work, and that anyway live donors within families would still need to be typed to discover *perfectly* matching kidneys. So he devised an ingenious way of keeping himself in business. Since 1967 he had been making a portable tissue-typing kit, giving it away to surgeons and others to let them do the matching themselves. To keep his laboratory afloat, Terasaki decided to sell the kits. In principle it was an excellent plan. There was just one problem: after withdrawing his funds, the National Institutes of Health started to make and give away the trays itself. 'So the Government gave them away free and we charged $15 for each tray. But we had enough people who had confidence in our tray to enable us to survive. We found we could get almost enough money by selling this tray as by having the grant! So we did OK. The tray sales kept going up – and the NIH ones kept going down. In the end they gave up. People were buying our tray rather than getting it free from the NIH because the quality of our tray was better.'

It was so good that eventually Terasaki's business was bringing in an annual income of $2 million – more than enough to keep his laboratory afloat and leave enough spare cash to buy him a mansion in Hollywood and a lifestyle more suited to a movie star than a medical researcher. 'I never would have thought things would come out like this, especially in 1970 when it seemed like all the work I had done was lost,' says Terasaki. '. . . When I look back to . . . the Hague meeting I see that I was quite naïve. I thought science was straightforward: that we look for the facts and describe them. But there is a lot more to it than that. Just telling how it was got me into a lot of trouble – a lot more than I ever expected.'

Terasaki's courage was costly, but his stand had a pivotal effect on transplant surgery at the beginning of the 1970s. It gave a new focus to those trying to find less harmful ways of preventing rejection. 'By exposing the truth,' says Tom Starzl, 'Terasaki had made it clear that the field of clinical transplantation could advance significantly only by the development of better drugs and other treatment strategies, not by vainly hoping that the solution would be through tissue matching.'[9]

There were only two other approaches to rejection. You could change the body in a way that made it less likely to attack a transplanted organ; this was the method adopted by those who had used X-rays or drugs to smother the body's immune defences. Or you could change the transplant itself, making it appear friend rather than foe to the army of white blood cells that would normally attack and destroy such an invader of bodily integrity. This was the Trojan Horse approach to transplantation, a technique that William Summerlin, a young American physician, stumbled across while working with burns patients at Stanford University Medical Centre near San Francisco. Summerlin thought he was on the trail of immunology's Holy Grail: a way of altering transplantable tissues and organs that would entirely prevent the destructive immune response. The body could be fooled, so he believed, into accepting the gift of life – and there would be no price to pay. Unlike all the other means of preventing rejection, his method appeared free of side effects. By 1971 Summerlin's work looked so promising that he was given his own laboratory at one of the country's leading research institutes, a staff of six medical researchers and a sizeable income of $50,000 a year. He suddenly found himself in the fast-lane, working at the cutting edge of immunological research on a technique that could transform transplant surgery and see his name placed alongside some of the great innovators of twentieth-century medicine. But three years later, Summerlin was disgraced, his career was in ruins and his name discredited. 'My interpretation was that he was totally obsessed with the enormous scientific implications. He just lost sight of the means,' says George Miller, one of Summerlin's former colleagues.

William Summerlin's doomed attempt to overcome rejection began with the best possible motive, the desire to save human life, and, as with many scientific discoveries, a chance observation. Summerlin wanted to help the badly burned patients with whom his work at Stanford University Medical Centre brought him into contact. The life of such patients literally drained out of their bodies, vital bodily fluids leaking from raw wounds. Bacteria, too, often found an easy entry-point, setting up infections that their injured bodies often could not fight off. One way of helping such patients over the crisis was to cover their burns with pigskin, in the knowledge that the tissue will eventually be rejected but hoping that it would buy sufficient time to overcome the initial devastating shock.

One of Summerlin's colleagues had developed a method of growing pig skin outside the body by incubating it in a nutrient fluid, when Summerlin began to wonder if human skin might provide a better stop-gap covering. In 1969 he seized an opportunity to test his idea.[10] 'I had a black man who I was grafting,' he says, 'and just happened to have some extra skin from a white patient that was left over in the incubator. And I decided to put it on a separate part of the wound . . . I wasn't going to hurt the patient, of course, and it wasn't a huge area . . . and, hell, it took just as well as the patient's own skin did. I thought: holy mackerel, that's just not supposed to be.'

It certainly wasn't. The laws of immunology said the donor's skin should have been rejected. The observation could, of course, have been a fluke, a one-in-a-million perfect match between the

donor and the recipient. So Summerlin did an experiment to see
if skin culturing really could prevent rejection. He took small
skin patches from volunteer donors, grew them in dishes for four
or five weeks, and then transplanted the patches onto four
unrelated patients. He expected the transplanted tissue to survive
about two weeks before it was rejected by its new host. In fact,
Summerlin reported, the transplants were not destroyed. They
were adopted by the patient's body as if they were their own
without the use of drugs to suppress the normal immune
reaction. This was a remarkable observation – particularly as it
involved the skin, a tissue that is usually rejected more fiercely
than any other organ in the body.[11] The ripples from
Summerlin's astonishing discovery spread rapidly through the
medical research world. If it was possible to prevent rejection
simply by growing tissues outside the body for a period of time,
the implications for transplantation were breathtaking. They
were just as intriguing for cancer research because the immune
system is also the body's first line of defence against cancer.
When news of Summerlin's work reached the ears of Robert
Good, the Regents Professor of Paediatrics and Microbiology at
the University of Minnesota, he reached for the phone. Good was
one of the country's top immunologists, with a formidable
intellect and a reputation to match. Since the 1960s, he had been
working at the cutting edge of transplant immunology, trying to
unravel the secrets of the human immune system in the hope of
solving these two riddles: the cause of rejection and the cause of
cancer. If Summerlin's work could be confirmed, Good thought
it could provide a crucial key, unlocking a much deeper level of
understanding of these mysterious processes. He asked him to
come to Minnesota to give his observations some scientific
backing.

Summerlin left Stanford in 1971 and started a series of
transplant experiments to see if he could reproduce the
phenomenon he had seen in his patients. He used mice, grafting
skin taken from one strain and cultured in laboratory dishes onto
the backs of a different strain. When Good left Minnesota to take
up a prestigious post as director of the Sloan-Kettering Institute,

the research arm of the Memorial Sloan-Kettering Cancer Centre in New York, he took his protégé with him.

In the space of a few months, William Summerlin's life had been transformed. From treating burns patients at a medical centre in Stanford, the thirty-three-year-old physician suddenly found himself in New York City at the hub of medical research. Good had made him the youngest full member of one of the top cancer-research centres in the country. He had bypassed the usual formalities and elevated Summerlin to a status that was the academic equivalent of being a full professor. He also appointed him head of the Memorial Hospital's skin-disease service. There was no doubt that William Summerlin had the director's ear – and no doubt either that the director had the highest hopes of Summerlin's research.

'When Summerlin came,' Good recalls, thinking back to the time when Summerlin first joined him in Minnesota, 'I took him out to my farm and we spent several days going over plans. When I had to go away during that period, Bill and his family stayed at the farm getting adjusted to Minnesota. I outlined the experiments that I thought would be necessary and that he ought to do. I helped him get oriented to the facilities and the people. I spent a great deal of time with him in those days . . . We were very close then.'[12]

At Sloan-Kettering, Summerlin expanded his efforts. He tried to transplant corneas taken from a number of different species after growing them in laboratory dishes, and did the same with adrenal glands taken from mice, and with skin taken from both humans and mice. By 1973 news of Summerlin's work began to reach a wider audience. His claims were dramatic and bold. 'I found that after human skin is maintained in organ culture for four to six weeks, it becomes universally transplantable without rejection,' he told the annual conference of American Cancer Society held in March of that year in Nogales, Arizona. 'Moreover work with other organs, including the mouse adrenal glands, shows that such organs maintain their function during organ culture and . . . function quite normally after such transplantation.'[13]

Summerlin's claims had a credibility and significance that they might not have achieved had they not had the backing of Robert Good, the immunologist with an international reputation, but because they were coming from so well-respected an institution as Sloan-Kettering, the American press sat up and took notice. 'Skin Graft Transplant Gain', read the headline in the *Kansas Star* after Summerlin's speech. 'Skin Banks May Some Day Aid Burn Victims' claimed the *Buffalo Evening News*, while the *New York Times* headline writer went for 'Lab Discovery May Aid Transplants'.

George Miller, a surgical ophthalmologist at the University of Minnesota, was so intrigued by Summerlin's work that he began a collaboration with him in culturing corneas to see if the technique really could prevent rejection. 'We felt with this research that we had a tiger by the tail,' he says. 'The idea that you could take an organ – a kidney, a heart from another animal species – and put it in some kind of a magical solution and . . . store it for just the right length of time so that the bad cells died and the good cells lived, and then be able to put that into the human body, that was an incredible thought . . . We felt that it was something that had enormous ability to influence the course of medicine. We felt it was so important that it probably would have been the type of discovery that would have been Nobel Prize calibre.'

In the two years that he had worked with Robert Good, Summerlin was attracting the kind of recognition that other medical researchers strive a life-time to achieve. But the publicity was double-edged. As news of his claims spread, medical researchers set out to confirm Summerlin's work – but no one was able to reproduce his astonishing results. The feedback that filtered up to Robert Good was uniformly bad. One letter that Sloan-Kettering's director received was from Leslie Brent, the English immunologist and one of the pioneers in the field of immunology. His experience was typical of many researchers who had delved into Summerlin's work.

'It seemed a very exciting possibility, unlikely but exciting,' Brent recalls, 'and I decided that I would try to repeat the work

. . . which depended on the culturing of skin two weeks before transplanting it to adult mice. And we did that and found that by the end of the two-week period the skin was actually dead and not really transplantable. The methods he had given in his papers were very inadequately described and you couldn't possibly follow the method exactly from his description. So I wrote to Summerlin and said, "Look, I'm trying to repeat this work, any possibility you could let me know what culture you used, [the] precise conditions, any problems." I didn't get a reply. And I wrote again and I still didn't get a reply. Eventually I became impatient and wrote to Robert Good.'

Brent wasn't the only academic with complaints to make to Good: Summerlin's own colleagues were finding themselves increasingly concerned by his claims and frustrated by his approach to the work. John Raaf, a postgraduate with a degree in biochemistry, had left Boston's Massachusetts General Hospital to do research at Sloan-Kettering. He was well used to the detailed demands of the scientific method and was greatly disturbed by his experience of working in Summerlin's laboratory. 'Summerlin always had great showmanship, but he did not have the scientific rigour I would have expected from someone in his position,' he says. 'There was a real show-business atmosphere in his lab, he was very enthusiastic, but when it came to the data . . . I think that many of us in the laboratory were always very unhappy about his approach to science . . . I was also looking at the effect of the culture on grafts, but the results that I was getting directly contradicted Summerlin's. I found that the culture technique had no effect. . . . Although I was working on different organs – I was working on the thyroid – I was finding the opposite results to Summerlin.'

Another disillusioned researcher was John Ninnemann, also a postgraduate on a temporary attachment to Summerlin's laboratory. His job was to duplicate the skin-culturing work on mice to provide scientific back-up for the Institute. 'It was a disaster,' he says. 'I had hoped that it would not take very long to confirm his observations. . . . I tried several different ways and spent a long time trying to replicate Summerlin's work, but I could not. So I took my results to Good. At that point I thought I was simply

missing something and I thought it was my own shortcoming so I
was not suspicious at all. Summerlin was a very charismatic figure
and he was a very hard worker.'

The doubters seemed to have little effect on Summerlin. In
May he told a meeting of the American Society for Clinical
Investigation in Atlantic City that cultured human corneas placed
in rabbits' eyes had survived for six months. This was an
astonishing claim. Transplants between different species always
elicit an extremely vigorous form of rejection and a six-month
survival of such a cross-species transplant was unheard-of. The
corneal transplants had been undertaken by two ophthalmolo-
gists from the Cornell-New York Hospital, Peter Laino and
Bartley Mondino. In October 1973, Summerlin presented two of
these transplanted rabbits to Sloan-Kettering's board of scientific
advisers, a group of eminent academics who meet periodically to
review the Institute's projects. Among the team was the British
zoologist Sir Peter Medawar, the 1960 Nobel Prize winner whose
work in the 1940s and 1950s had laid the foundation stone of
transplantation immunology. Summerlin held up his rabbits for
inspection and told the board that one eye in each of the animals
had been transplanted with a human cornea grown in the
laboratory for several weeks. The other eye, he explained, had
been grafted with a freshly removed human cornea. Sir Peter and
the rest of the board of advisers took turns to peer closely at the
rabbits' eyes. They saw one cloudy cornea that had obviously been
rejected by the rabbit's immune system and one normally
functioning transparent one. Summerlin proclaimed that the
clear corneas were the ones that he had cultured in dishes before
stitching them into the rabbits' eyes.

John Ninnemann was also at the meeting and was puzzled by
this claim. He had recently spoken with Mondino who had told
him quite clearly that they had only ever transplanted fresh
corneas into one eye in each rabbit. At the time of the meeting of
the board of advisers, Mondino told Ninnemann, they hadn't yet
used any cultured ones. 'So here was Dr Summerlin,' says
Ninnemann, 'showing a rabbit's eye that hadn't been grafted at all
and saying it was an example of how cultured cornea wouldn't be

rejected like a fresh cornea. So I confronted Dr Summerlin on this and he said: 'No, no. I'm sure you're mistaken. I know they were grafted on both sides. Let's go up to the animal room and I'll show you.' So we went through every cage there and we could not find any animal in which both sides had been grafted.'[14]

After this incident Ninnemann asked Robert Good to transfer him away from Summerlin to another laboratory. Good certainly had ample cause for worry. In January 1974, he was expecting a site visit from the National Institutes of Health to help them decide whether to fund Summerlin's immunology research to the tune of over $600,000 over the next five years. He needed the kind of unambiguous results that Summerlin appeared to be getting at Minnesota, but all he heard was criticism. In the circumstances, his protégé's performance at a review meeting two months before the visit was all the more mystifying.

'When he made his presentation,' Good says, 'I was just dumbfounded. He didn't present any of the questions that were being raised. He just presented it as though it was the same as the spring before, without any of the failures Ninnemann and Raaf were getting. I talked to him. I said, "Gee, Bill, it's just as though Brent didn't exist, as though Ninnemann didn't exist." And he said, "I am absolutely convinced that these are all technical matters." . . . There have been many examples of investigators, particularly after they have changed locations, failing to duplicate previous findings. That's why I didn't dump the Summerlin thing in the winter of 1973.'[15]

By January, Summerlin's claims to have successfully crossed the species barrier with cultured corneal transplants came under further fire. The ophthalmologist Peter Laino had grafted cultured human corneas into the eyes of twenty rabbits at the New York Hospital without a single success. 'It appears that no appreciable difference in acceptance or rejection time occurs when these eyes are compared to others grafted directly into recipients without having first been passed through tissue culture,' he wrote in a letter to Summerlin. 'They both fail at about the same time.'[16]

William Summerlin was under considerable pressure. The NIH

scientists who had visited his laboratory in January had not been impressed. He had shown them various animals that, he said, were thriving with cultured organs inside them. Among them were rabbits with human corneas in one of their eyes and the 'Old Man', a brown mouse that had had a patch of skin from a white mouse transplanted onto its back, according to Summerlin, three years earlier. But it wasn't enough. The NIH turned down Summerlin's grant application. In March they agreed to reconsider their decision – but by then Robert Good wanted some clear answers to the mounting criticism. He summoned Summerlin to a 7 a.m. meeting in his office on the thirteenth floor of the Kettering Laboratory.

About half an hour before the meeting, Summerlin made his way up to the eleventh floor of Kettering's Howard Laboratory, just across the street from Good's office. He went into the Institute's animal quarters and selected two of his best-looking grafted mice to show to Good. They were white and carried skin transplanted from black mice on their backs. Summerlin placed the two animals into a metal container, carried them into the lift and pressed the button to take him down to street level. On the way down he took one of the mice out of its container and inspected the graft on its back. Skin cells that are cultured outside the body have a tendency to lose their colour and the patches of transplanted skin, which should have been black, had taken on a dirty grey hue. Summerlin then did something he would later regret. He took a felt-tip pen out of the breast pocket of his white coat and inked in the patches, restoring to them something like the dark colour they had once had. He repeated the operation on the other mouse and then took them up to Robert Good's office in time for his early-morning meeting.

Perhaps Good was too preoccupied with his worries about Summerlin's work, but the director did not notice the ink that clearly distinguished the transplanted patches on Summerlin's mice from the rest of the skin on their backs. But Summerlin's laboratory assistant spotted it when he was handed the mice after the meeting. James Martin was about to replace the two animals in their cages when he noticed the unusually dark patches on their backs. Curious, he soaked some cotton in alcohol and rubbed it against the transplanted skin. The cotton turned black – and a few hours later Summerlin's face turned red when Good confronted him with the evidence.

'This was the first time that I really doubted Summerlin's veracity,' says Good. 'There had been plenty of problems about the science, but this was the first time I had doubted Summerlin's honesty. Right then, a kaleidoscope of questions went through my mind about the mice with guinea-pig skin grafts that had been prolonged and the white skin on the brown mice that he had showed us before, all the grafts he had presented to us in the past. I realized that no matter how closely I could have watched, I could have been fooled.'[17]

Science moves forward in a slow but methodical way. Its power is derived from the repeatability of its discoveries. One researcher's claims must be reproduced in other laboratories before they can be accepted into the growing body of scientific knowledge. No one expects researchers to be right all the time but they must be honest. Truth is the bedrock of the scientific method and Summerlin's decision to ink in the transplanted skin on the backs of his mice had contravened this most basic of principles. News of the deception fell like a bombshell on his professional colleagues.

'I was very shocked and quite disappointed,' says John Ninnemann. 'I was in a fast-lane research environment which was very new to me and this was really a great opportunity for me to be working with such great people. I expected all of the good things and it was a kind of nasty surprise to find out . . . I had had such high expectations at that time.'

John Raaf was equally upset. 'I was just devastated,' he says. 'I was very young at that time and very idealistic about science . . . but it was kind of consistent with his approach of not being too careful with the accuracy of data. So although we were unhappy with the rigorousness of his data, we had not suspected that he was actually misrepresenting something to that degree.'

In March 1974 William Summerlin was suspended from his post at the Sloan-Kettering Institute. An official investigation held two months later was a scathing indictment of his scientific approach. The committee wanted Summerlin to show them some of the mice he claimed to have successfully transplanted with cultured skin. But the only mouse he could produce was the 'Old Man', which Summerlin claimed bore skin on its back that had been transplanted more than two years ago. The rest of his supposedly successful brood had been killed at intervals, he explained, to obtain serum for a special test. Summerlin had sacrificed the animals on which his credibility rested and the investigators were understandably perplexed. 'It is scarcely conceivable,' they wrote in their report, 'that Dr Summerlin could have believed . . . that it is necessary to kill a mouse to obtain serum.'[18] Instead of the mice, the investigators looked at the statistics that he had used to claim success in an article in the respected *Journal of Experimental Medicine*. They asked him what criteria he had used in working out the figures quoted in the paper for the percentage of grafts that had been accepted on his mice. 'Dr Summerlin gave no coherent reply,' the investigation concluded, 'and implied that even a few days of prolonged graft survival under ill-defined conditions might be considered a "success".'

The only living proof of the success of his culturing technique was the 'Old Man' mouse. But even that claim was demolished by a simple test proving that the animal was a hybrid (mixed breed) rather than a pure-bred animal. It was, in short, genetically contaminated and the survival of the 'Old Man's' graft could be easily explained by well-understood genetic laws rather than the effects of Summerlin's culturing technique.

Summerlin did not dispute the felt-tip-pen incident. He called it an 'unthinkable act' brought about by what he called the 'extreme personal and professional stress' he was feeling. 'I guess if you hadn't been there you just can't ever know,' he says. '[It was] just monstrous – monstrous pressure because, as it turns out, a lot of investigatory monetary support was linked into some of the work that I was doing and so the need for good data to keep the money flowing was very real.' As for the rabbits, Summerlin explained his mistaken belief that both their eyes had been

transplanted by saying that he had been unable to contact either
Dr Laino or Dr Mondino to check this. The committee dismissed
this out of hand. 'The necessary information could have been
obtained within a day or so at the longest, either personally or by
note-of-hand, or by a call to the private residence of Dr Laino or
Dr Mondino. The only possible conclusion is that Dr Summerlin
was responsible for initiating and perpetuating a profound and
serious misrepresentation about the results of transplanting
cultured human corneas to rabbits.'

The committee condemned William Summerlin for indulging
in irresponsible conduct incompatible with his scientific respon-
sibilities. 'Fellow investigators,' they wrote in their report, 'are
justified in assuming that pronouncements of new observations
by other scientists are made on the basis of adequate data,
systematically obtained, recorded and interpreted according to
accepted standards of investigation; since this is evidently not the
case with Dr Summerlin's experiments with mice it is the opinion
of the committee that he has propagated misconceptions
concerning the nature and scope of his work in this area.'

Summerlin was sacked. Robert Good was rebuked for failing to
act soon enough on his doubts and for not consulting with his
colleagues before promoting Summerlin to such a senior post in
the Institute. 'It had tremendous negative consequences for my
career,' says Good. 'It was argued that I had fostered someone
who had falsified and faked scientific data and that is the worst
offence that a scientist can commit. The rules of the game are that
you have to record faithfully what you have observed. He broke
every rule. It really made my work much more difficult.'

But can Summerlin pin the blame for this sorry story on
mental exhaustion and pressure of work? His former colleagues
have other ideas about the cause of this scientific catastrophe. 'He
was really on a high,' says George Miller, an ophthalmologist at
the University of Minnesota who had collaborated with Summerlin and tried to confirm the results of his cross-species corneal
transplants. 'It may have been that he had done some initial
research and got some good results and was so swept away with
the enormous implications for humankind that he lost his

perspective. He was totally swept up in the work that he was doing. . . . He just lost sight of the means.'

The real loser in all this was transplantation itself. Even the investigating committee recognized that some of the work Summerlin was doing might have had some merit – particularly his use of cultured human skin.[19] But this line of research was dropped like a hot potato in the aftermath of the scandal.

'Of course he did something very foolish,' says John Ninnemann. 'But the original observation that he made claim to was never really explained . . . Following the scandal, the work on culturing was abandoned because the whole thing was such a terrible event. It became an area of research that no one wanted to touch. It was one area which caused all those concerned nothing but pain. It is possible that there are beneficial results from the culture for grafting – but the players had had enough and they just did not want to know any more.'[20]

The Summerlin affair had jeopardized the good reputation of the Sloan-Kettering Institute and its talented director – and had brought to an early end the career of a young man who once thought he held the key to the future of transplant surgery. William Summerlin is now a dermatologist caring for patients in a medical centre in Rogers, Arkansas. There was, however, one positive outcome, for the scandal at least refocused the fight against rejection. If transplants could not be altered to prevent the body from attacking them, and if our knowledge of tissue typing needed to grow before the system could be made to work, then drugs were the only weapons left in the surgeon's arsenal. The failure of Summerlin's mice and rabbits to deliver the solution to rejection had only served to highlight the crying need for a more selective means of persuading the body to accept the gift of life.

What few realized at the height of the row at Sloan-Kettering was that a real breakthrough had just been made in a laboratory in Switzerland. It was a drug that would revolutionize transplant surgery, offering new hope to patients suffering the debilitating side effects of steroids and giving fresh confidence to surgeons wanting to add the lung, the stomach, the intestines, and other organs to the list of life-saving transplants. It would be hailed as a wonder drug, but before the cork could be pulled out of the champagne bottle, the company that had discovered the chemical threatened to drop it. They thought it would be too expensive to test and develop.

If you were to look inside the suitcases carried by employees of the giant Swiss pharmaceutical firm Sandoz while on foreign holidays or business trips, as likely as not you would find a collection of small plastic bags filled with a dark crumbly material. At first glance, you could be forgiven for jumping to the conclusion that these drug-company executives were indulging in a little illegal pharmaceutical recreation. You would be wrong, of course: the plastic bags might indeed contain powerful chemicals but, far from being illegal, they would be as yet undiscovered drugs hidden in soil samples that Sandoz employees frequently collect while travelling abroad. Since 1958, Sandoz has been screening such soil samples in the hope of discovering new medicines that, once tested, packaged and marketed, would add to the company's already sizeable assets. It was in one such soil sample, brought back from the Hardanger Vidda in Norway in 1969, that the drug that would change the face of transplant surgery was found. Sandoz regularly checked soil samples for compounds with antibacterial or antifungal properties. But it was only in 1966, as transplant surgery was beginning to get off the ground, that they began to check for chemicals that might affect the immune system. They did this at an industrial estate on the outskirts of Basle where the company owned a large building containing experimental laboratories. The immunology laboratory was led by a microbiologist called Hartmann Stähelin, who had developed the test for immuno-suppressive compounds; his chemists regularly checked about a thousand substances each year for their ability to prevent rejection. A fungus extracted from the Norwegian soil sample, and known unromantically as 24-556, was delivered into his laboratory around Christmas 1971.

'They gave it to our laboratory without knowing what it could do so it went into the screening system,' says Stähelin. 'The first person who noticed it was a technician called Sibylle Stutz. She put the result into a form and then it came to me.' Stutz had noted on the test form that the substance appeared to have a 'very marked' ability to depress the immune system.

This was a rare observation and Stähelin sat up and took notice. 'Such a strong reduction of the immune response had not been found many times before,' he says, 'but I also knew from very long experience that it's sometimes impossible to repeat many of the results in a screening because there has been some mistake or for a number of other reasons. So before I made a big fuss, I wanted to be sure the result was correct.'

His caution was not misplaced. The drug's powerful impact on the immune system mysteriously vanished when it was tested again on mice. Stähelin wasn't satisfied. Surely, he thought, such a marked effect could not have been a mere fluke? Eventually he discovered the problem: the solution into which 24-556 had been dissolved before it was given to the mice played a crucial part in determining whether or not it was absorbed into the animal's body. In the first test, they had dissolved it in water to which they had added two chemicals (dimethyl sulphoxide and sorbitan monoleate) and it had worked. In the second, they'd tried to dissolve it in pure water and it had not. It was a simple solution. But if it hadn't been found, the drug that was soon to revolutionize transplant surgery might have been ignored. Further tests proved the value of 24-556, and by the time Summerlin was being drummed out of the Sloan-Kettering Institute, some of Stähelin's natural Swiss reserve began to vanish. 'When I saw the results . . . and saw that we had got such a strong effect, it was clear then that I could get excited,' he explains. 'What we had found was new. Before this there had not been an immuno-suppressant that did not damage the bone marrow.'

By 1976, it was clear that mushroom sample 24-556 was a new and powerful immuno-suppressant agent. It was time to convince the wider world of its value, and Jean Borel, an immunologist at Sandoz who had conducted some of the animal tests on the compound, travelled to London in April to spread the good news at the congress of the British Society of Immunology. At the meeting, Borel met two Englishmen with a particular interest in the mysterious mushroom: Roy (now Sir Roy) Calne, the transplant surgeon who fifteen years earlier had been the first to show that drugs could prevent rejection,[21] and David White, the immunologist from Cambridge.

The new compound was in short supply, but by 1977 White had obtained enough of it to begin his own animal tests.[22] The results were startling: transplanted rats lived nearly five times as long with the new drug. 'I can remember the precise moment that I discussed these results with Roy Calne,' says White, 'because I had made an appointment to see him and his secretary said he wasn't there, he was on the ward. So I went to find him and he was sitting in one of the patients' rooms watching Chris Evert play Virginia Wade in the semi-finals at Wimbledon. He looked at those results and said he didn't trust the data and told me to go away and do them again.'

There was no mistake. The new drug, now called Cyclosporin A, appeared to be better at preventing rejection than anything else in the immunologists' armoury. Calne wanted to test it on larger animals but had only a small supply of the substance. He rang Sandoz and asked for some more, only to be told something that he didn't want to hear. 'They said they'd stopped working with the drug,' Sir Roy recalls. 'Well, I was extremely anxious that we should develop it because it seemed so much better than anything that we'd had before.'

The problem was simple: money. Putting a new drug on the market is an expensive, risky business and, in the beginning, the drug proved difficult to produce in large enough quantities – and even more difficult to purify. 'If you use a drug it has to be pure,' says Jean Borel, 'and while you could produce a 98 per cent pure drug like Cyclosporin in the laboratory, you could not produce it by the tonne as it would be needed. The fungus doesn't just contain Cyclosporin A, it contains a lot of different cyclosporins which are not necessarily immuno-suppressive but which almost all behave physically alike. Therefore new technology had to be made to produce it in large quantities.'

It might cost up to $500 million to get a new drug out of the laboratory and into the clinic. Safety testing is also costly, and Sandoz thought the transplant market too small to warrant such a huge outlay. At a time when only the kidney was routinely being transplanted, this was understandable. But the men who took the financial decisions at Sandoz missed the wider picture. They didn't see that a new, powerful immuno-suppressant might create the very market they needed to justify their development costs. Sandoz's scientists, however, realized the drug's potential and devised a nifty plan to keep the project alive. The drug had also shown some promise as an anti-inflammatory agent so they recategorized it to keep Calne supplied with enough Cyclosporin for his tests. 'We ran out of the substance and needed official permission in order to produce more of it,' explains Borel. 'To get that permission we had to say it was anti-inflammatory.'

Calne tested the drug on larger animals, with spectacular results. It doubled the survival time of dogs'[23] with kidney transplants, compared to those given existing treatments for rejection. It was even more effective when used on pigs with transplanted hearts. On average they survived ten times as long as animals given Imuran and steroid treatment.[24]

Cyclosporin, however, needed Sandoz's full backing if it was ever going to get off the ground as an anti-rejection drug rather than as an anti-inflammatory agent. There were still too many doubters on the board of management among those who counted, so Jean Borel asked Calne and White to fly to Switzerland to convince the sceptics that it was worth the investment. He knew that Calne's views, in particular, would carry weight with his management committee: it had been Calne, after all, who had pioneered the use of drugs to combat rejection, and by the mid 1970s he had a wealth of clinical experience of transplantation that could not be lightly dismissed. In November 1977 the two Englishmen flew to Basle on a mission to rescue a drug that they believed could transform the face of transplant surgery.

'We more or less had to sell them their own drug,' remembers David White. 'It was all big mahogany tables, cigars, Swiss accountants. I presented the technical data to them, Roy presented the world view about transplantation. At that stage they knew nothing about it. Of course, in those days transplantation meant kidney transplantation. There were one or two brave souls doing liver transplants and one brave soul doing heart transplants – but that was all. Jean Borel said: "Look. Even if you don't make any money, transplantation is a high-profile activity, so it will be like a loss leader and Sandoz's name will be to the forefront." And I think that was the selling point. They all went off in a conflab after a whole day of this and decided to put their high risk money into Cyclosporin. We'd sold it to them.'

Jean Borel breathed a deep sigh of relief. He had put his reputation on the line: 'It was very unusual – even revolutionary – to convene such a conference where a lab person like me was asking management to meet scientists and be persuaded by something I was convinced of,' he says. 'So I was extremely relieved when in the evening they thanked me and said, yes, they will continue to develop Cyclosporin. This was really a great event for me.'

The manufacture of Cyclosporin proved as difficult as Borel had feared, but when it was first tried out in patients, the results more than made up for the problems. Roy Calne began using it to prevent rejection in kidney-transplant recipients at Addenbrooke's Hospital in Cambridge in June 1978. Four months later, he presented his results at a meeting of the Transplantation Society in Rome.

'Rumours flew that sensational findings would be disclosed,' remembers Jean Borel, 'and the small room was soon overcrowded with still more people spilling into the hallway to hear [the] results . . . His oral report was a milestone: it showed that Cyclosporin alone effectively prevented rejection in patients and ushered in a gold rush for the new compound. A new era in transplantation had begun.'[25]

Cyclosporin is so effective because it is highly selective, only hitting a small proportion of the white blood cells, those that are responsible for destroying transplanted organs. This means that it can prevent rejection without also opening the patient to overwhelming infection. By the early 1980s, transplant surgeons began to clamour for the new drug. 'It was crazy because everybody wanted to use it,' says David White. 'Poor old Sandoz couldn't produce it fast enough. They were completely taken by surprise . . . What Cyclosporin did was to turn a narrow tightrope into a fairly broad plank. There are still risks from infection. There are still rejection episodes, but what it has done is make them much much less ferocious. In the old days the kidney would swell up, the patient would get a fever. I think about 60 per cent of our kidney patients would stop passing urine from the transplant. You rarely see that nowadays. It's quite mild and readily treatable.'

With such a powerful and selective anti-rejection drug to call on in their battle against the immune system, surgeons began to transplant organs like the lungs, which would have been considered far too risky before the days of Cyclosporin. Ron Grundon, from Ventura in California, would not be alive today but for the discovery of Cyclosporin. He was born with a hole in his heart and, by the time he was old enough to benefit from an operation, his lungs had been hopelessly damaged by high blood pressure. A few lung transplants had been attempted before the discovery of Cyclosporin, but with little success. Infection or rejection had killed the few patients who had had the operation, but for Ron Grundon, confined to a wheelchair, unable even to get dressed without the assistance of his wife, such an operation was his only hope of staying alive. 'I was continually short of breath,' he explains. 'I would gasp for air putting on my socks. Anything like that was a major exertion. My heart would sometimes start beating real irregular and I'd just reach up and thump my heart like this [he demonstrates, hitting his chest]. I didn't know why it would work but it would put it back in synch and stop the quivering feeling that I'd had.'

Grundon's doctor had told him that medical science could do nothing for him, that surgeons were not offering lung transplants because they had proved so unsuccessful. His advice was that Ron Grundon should go home, write a will and get ready to die. Then, in October 1981, he read an article about a journalist, dying of lung disease who had been offered a lung transplant because she had managed to get a supply of Cyclosporin before its formal approval for clinical use. She had survived the operation. 'The article that I saw talked specifically about Cyclosporin,' Grundon says. 'It also said that she had pulmonary hypertension and I knew that was exactly what my problem was. So when I saw this I really got hope then.'

In March 1982 Ron Grundon was put on the waiting list for a transplant at Stanford University Medical Centre. Two months later he received a new heart and lungs. His first memory after waking up from the anaesthetic was of the colour of his body. 'I was amazed,' he says. 'Before I went to sleep I was blue – my face and lips and fingernails were always blue. But when I woke my fingernails were pink. A few hours later I looked in the mirror and saw that my lips and face were pink. So that was how I knew that I had had the surgery . . . being able to breathe again like that. I felt totally natural.'

Ron Grundon is now the longest surviving heart-lung recipient in the world. From being a wheelchair cripple facing certain death, he has now enjoyed fourteen years of good health that would have been impossible without Cyclosporin. His success story has since been mirrored in thousands of other transplant patients given new leases on life by the drug.

'I think it changed transplantation from a rather crazy endeavour by a few misguided surgeons who were getting some good results . . . into a form of treatment . . . for many otherwise fatal diseases,' says Sir Roy Calne, 'not just kidney disease, but also heart disease, liver disease, lung disease and diabetes. So for the first time transplantation was being sought as a form of treatment in a world-wide manner instead of by a few people in special conditions and often regarded in a cynical way by some of the people who weren't doing transplantation. So it did completely transform the field.'

Cyclosporin was not the perfect answer to rejection. It had some side effects and sometimes failed to keep the immune system muzzled. But it rapidly became the mainstay of transplant surgery. Before the introduction of the drug, only 55 per cent of kidney-transplant patients were still alive one year after their operations. With Cyclosporin in the early 1980s this figure climbed to 85 per cent.[26] Heart and liver transplantation began to come in from the cold, increasingly recognized as a practical therapy for inoperable diseases of these organs, and surgeons successfully transplanted organs like the small bowel and the pancreas, which had been considered untransplantable before the discovery of Cyclosporin.

Throughout the 1980s, transplant surgery was frequently making headlines: a mercy flight for a life-saving transplant; a new longevity record; the almost magical restoration of a child's health and vitality. Such stories made good copy and even better news pictures. But the doctors' success with Cyclosporin was double-edged. Demand for organs burgeoned until the desperately sick were queuing for the chance of life. For some, that chance never came: they died on the waiting list. It was ironic that just as the transplanters began to get the science right, they started to run out of organs.

6

Dying for an Organ

Rustin Morris was in his early twenties and had suffered from cystic fibrosis, the lung disease, since he was six. He had been in and out of hospital more times than he could count with chest infections that most of us would shrug off without a second thought. To Rustin's weakened lungs, though, they were life-threatening episodes. 'When I have a chest infection I'm pretty much wheelchair-bound,' he said. 'I can't walk very far before I become extremely breathless because you bring up an awful lot of thick secretions off your chest. You're coughing, spluttering and I need oxygen given to me all the time. Any sort of exercise is out of the question. My appetite decreases massively – weight loss.'

Intravenous drugs and intensive physiotherapy kept Rustin alive. But it was a downhill slope. Even when he was well, he still needed oxygen at night, dispensed from a special machine installed in his flat in the Isle of Wight. His illness forced him to abandon a university degree course after three years of studying. He knew he was not going to get any better – and so did his doctors, who placed him on the waiting list for a heart-lung transplant. 'To put it bluntly, without the transplant, the prognosis isn't particularly marvellous,' said Rustin, from a hospital bed where he is recovering from another infection. 'I don't know what the time limit is on it but over the last two years the visits to hospital have become a lot more regular and the infections have become harder and harder to shift – until you have a particularly bad infection which you can't ever shake off and then it's just a matter of time before you die.'

Rustin Morris never had his transplant. Just a few weeks after voicing his thoughts, he succumbed to the illness that had plagued his life. His doctor couldn't find a suitable organ in time to save his life.

Today there are thousands of desperately ill people in a similar predicament. A transplant could end their suffering tomorrow but instead of a cure they are offered the torment of a lottery. Every day that passes on the waiting list is a day nearer the moment when they will be too sick to benefit from the operation. It is a cruel fate for people whose illnesses have already caused them so much suffering. The statistics make depressing reading: in 1994, 50,000 US citizens, more than 40,000 people in Western Europe and over 100,000 Asians were languishing on transplant waiting lists. Many never make it. About 5 per cent of patients waiting for new kidneys and between 15 and 25 per cent of those queuing for other organs die before they can be transplanted.[1] It is intensely frustrating for doctors, who know that they have the skill to save their lives but lack the raw materials. The shortage of donors forces transplant surgeons to play God with their patients: choosing life for some and death for others.

'Making choices is difficult and you can't pretend it doesn't exist,' says John Wallwork, the surgeon at Papworth Hospital in Cambridge who would have operated on Rustin Morris had a lung become available in time. 'How do you choose? Do you choose the person you're about to see? Do you choose the person who's going to contribute most to society? Do you choose the person who's the youngest? Do you choose the person who's got the wherewithal to pay? Do you choose the person who you regard as worthy – so do you do bishops and dons and not pop stars and pimps? It's a complicated issue as to who you choose. Medicine is a process of learning how to agonize without destroying yourself.'

Many people are never accepted onto the waiting list. They are rejected because they have another disease like cancer, because they are too old or simply too weak to stand the rigours of the operation. Once a patient is accepted, the choice of who gets the organs that become available is not a simple matter of first come, first served. Force of circumstance frequently determines this decision. 'We tend to take the person who is the sickest,' explains John Wallwork. 'That seems to be the right thing to do because, theoretically, the person who is the least sick can wait the longest. Often we are confined by time, so we take the person who's the nearest. If we are phoned at midnight and told there's a lung coming out somewhere and you can have it in a couple of hours, we don't tend to bring somebody in from Northern Ireland for that.'

The problem facing doctors in all countries that have a transplant service is the need to take organs from the bodies of people who have just been declared dead. There are too few live donors willing to donate organs, and grieving relatives must be asked at an intensely distressing time if they will let the death of their loved one bring life to someone else. More than a third of relatives still refuse permission.

'I believe it's because there is a feeling that it is a violation of the body in some way – the image of having a loved one cut up,' says Paddy Yeoman, a consultant in intensive care at Queen's Medical Centre in Nottingham. 'A lot of people find this very difficult to imagine. It is pretty horrific in fact. There's a feeling of protection towards the body, partly because a lot of the people who die are so young. They imagine them being cut through the chest, things being hacked out. It's a very emotional feeling. I'm amazed so many people do consent to be honest. I normally make the point that they would be stitched up very carefully, and the eyes would be closed afterwards so the body will be kept as dignified as possible.'

Many attempts have been made to increase the supply of organs: governments run publicity campaigns that extol the virtues of transplantation; donor cards make it easy to identify volunteers; bodies such as Eurotransplant have been set up to co-ordinate the exchange of organs and encourage transplantation. But none of these measures has worked. The supply of transplantable organs is still erratic: in the five European countries covered by Eurotransplant (Austria, Belgium, Germany, Luxembourg and The Netherlands) for example, the number of 'brain-dead' increased by 5 per cent in 1993; slumped by 10 per cent in the year after that and rose again by 2.5 per cent in 1995.

The most radical means of increasing the supply in Western nations is the 'opt-out' system, in which doctors can remove the organs of a brain-dead individual without the need to consult relatives. They can presume that a potential donor has consented

to the removal of their organs unless they have stated otherwise
(in a register kept specially for the purpose) during their lifetime.
More organs are donated in Austria, Belgium and Finland, which
have all introduced the opt-out system, than in countries that
practise informed consent (where doctors have to get the
permission of relatives before removing organs).[2] 'Presumed
consent' is controversial. Its opponents, and there are many in the
medical profession, believe it undermines basic notions of civil
liberty. In Spain, for example, doctors have simply ignored the
opt-out legislation introduced by their governments, their desire
to respect the dead and not to offend distressed relatives putting a
brake on attempts to use the law to increase the supply of organs.[3]
France also introduced opt-out laws, but here the system caused a
political storm when the parents of a young man killed in a road
accident complained that doctors had disfigured their son by
removing his eyes, one organ that they were not permitted to
remove without consent. The case became a *cause célèbre*: doctors
were accused of letting their concern for the living undermine
their respect for the dead.

'Our son was a person,' says Mireille Tesniere, the young man's
mother, 'but the doctors thought of him as a thing. Organs are
things. The doctors wouldn't do to their own child what they did
to Christophe.'

On Sunday 28 July 1991, Christophe Tesniere was cycling
home in the northern French town of Dieppe when he was
knocked off his bike by a passing motorist and suffered a crushing
blow to his head. The nineteen-year-old was rushed to the local
hospital with injuries so severe that his breathing failed. To keep
him alive, doctors placed him on a ventilator and three days later
flew him sixty miles by helicopter to the University Hospital of
North Amiens, which is better equipped to care for patients with
serious head injuries. A week later Christophe's parents, Alain
and Mireille Tesniere, were ushered into a small office in the
hospital's neurosurgery department to be told that their hopes for
the recovery of their son were in vain. Dr Jean Tchaoussoff, the
man in charge of the neurosurgical intensive care unit, said that
Christophe's brain was dead: it showed no electrical activity. Once

the ventilator was switched off, their son's heart would soon cease to pump blood round his body.

As well as being the department's unit chief, Tchaoussoff was also the president of the northern section of France Transplant[4] and, once he had broken the tragic news to the Tesnieres, he asked them whether Christophe had ever expressed the desire to be an organ donor. 'We had never discussed this idea,' says Alain. 'Why should a young man who is in good health think about his death? Why should he expect to die in five minutes by crossing a road? So we did not know.'

Tchaoussoff then asked Alain and Mireille their opinion of organ donation. Legally, due to the opt-out law, there was no need for Tchaoussoff to make this request – but, as a matter of courtesy, doctors tended to consult relatives if they could find them. Alain Tesniere had always supported organ donation, and had recently been moved by a TV programme about a young boy on the waiting list for a transplant, so he raised no objections.

Mireille, however, wanted to know which organs would be taken and says she asked for reassurance about the extent of the disfigurement that the removals would cause. Her son's body had already been badly damaged in the accident and she didn't want to add to the mutilation. She says the doctor asked for four organs: Christophe's heart, his liver and both his kidneys, and that he assured the parents that their son's body would otherwise be left alone. Mireille was content with his explanation and the parents gave their agreement for the doctors to remove four organs.

The trouble began with an accounting error. The Tesnieres received a bill from the University Hospital of South Amiens (where Christophe's organs were removed) asking for 300 francs to cover the cost of their son's hospitalization. It should not have been sent to them and they received an apology. But the damage was done: on the accounting form was a list detailing which organs had been taken. It was in code but its length puzzled them. The Tesnieres had agreed to the removal of four organs, but the list contained more. They asked for an explanation and found that surgeons had not only taken the heart, the liver and the two kidneys, but had also removed veins and arteries from

Christophe's legs and, worst of all for the distressed mother and father, both of his eyes so that his corneas might be used to restore someone's sight.

Christophe Tesniere's body was still in the hospital mortuary when his parents discovered the extent to which it had been emptied of its organs. Alain's visit to the hospital to say goodbye to his son before he was buried turned into a nightmare when he saw that Christophe's eyes had been replaced by what he describes as oversized glass ones. 'When I think about Christophe,' he says bitterly, 'I can't remember him as he was when he was living. It's a frightful thing not to have a memory of my son. I remember his eyes, those terrible eyes. It's like a second death.'

Mireille was just as angry at what she saw as a violation of her son's body. 'They stole our memory of Christophe,' she says. 'We had implicitly refused to donate his eyes. For us they were the symbol of life, much more important than any other organ.'[5]

The Amiens affair, as it came to be known, blew up into a major row. The Tesnieres took their distress to the press, gave endless interviews to the newspapers and on television. They wrote to the health minister asking for an enquiry into organ transplantation. Alain Tesniere even wrote a book. The effect of the publicity on the kidney-transplant service was disastrous.

'Immediately afterwards, there was a dramatic drop in organ donations of 20 per cent,' says Dr Philippe Romano, at L'Etablissement Français des Greffes, the organization that has now replaced France Transplant. 'This has not picked up, it has still dropped by 10 per cent. It was obviously not just due to the Tesnieres, but this dramatic story put a spotlight on this problem. In people's minds, there has been a loss of confidence with medicine in general and with medical people.'

The Tesnieres also consulted a lawyer who discovered that the doctors who removed their son's eyes might have broken the law, despite the existence of France's 'opt out' system. The reason was an oversight in the drafting of the Caillavet Law that introduced the presumed consent system of organ donation in 1976. This law did indeed permit the removal of organs from a brain-dead body without the need to consult with relatives. But it said nothing specifically about the corneas – and there was another statute dating back to 1949 called the Lafay Law which said that corneas could *only* be removed if a dead person had agreed to this in writing in their will. The cornea was an exception to the 'opt out' system. So in 1992 the Tesnieres decided to bring a prosecution against the doctors, charging them with theft and violation of their son's body.

'There was a contradiction between the two laws, a legal gap,' explains Professor Didier Houssin, the director-general of L'Etablissement Français des Greffes. 'It led to the ability to build a legal case . . . and it also showed the limits of what is tolerable in terms of multi-tissue harvesting. There has been a tendency to harvest many organs and tissues, to think: "While we are here we will take everything." It is an easy option but it has very negative aspects. It is a practical attitude which can be perceived by outsiders as a lack of respect, even if that wasn't the intention of the doctors.'

Tchaoussoff says the Lafay Law was written before people's bodies could be kept alive artificially on ventilators. He believes it does not apply to brain-dead bodies and, given the existence of the opt-out legislation, he does not accept that he overstepped the mark. 'If I didn't mention taking out Christophe's eyes to his parents, it's partly because it is not always technically possible to do it,' he says, 'but also because it is a particularly difficult thing to speak about with families.'[6]

The Tesnieres are still pursuing their legal case against the transplant doctors in Amiens. The damaging row also helped to bring about a fundamental reassessment of the French approach to organ donation. The 1976 Caillavet Law was a product of the political philosophy current in France in the 1970s in which the family took second place to the needs of society. Patients in need of organs were given a higher priority than the feelings of the families of potential donors. 'If the family happened to be present and expressed the deceased's opinion, saying no or yes, that was good,' says Professor Houssin. 'But it was not obligatory for the doctor to approach the family. This was the 1976 law.

The idea was to avoid imposing the burden of the decision onto the family.'

The Tesniere case also highlighted a major problem with presumed consent: there was no practical, foolproof way of making your views about organ donation known during your lifetime. 'If someone wanted to prevent their organs being taken,' Houssin continues, 'they had to sign a register at the entrance of the hospital. In fact, this was practically impossible for if you arrive at the hospital brain-dead or nearly brain-dead, you are in no condition to sign anything. This hadn't been clearly thought out.'

The Catholic Church also waded into the fray, letting it be known that it felt that the balance between the needs of society and the rights of the family had swung too far in favour of the community. 'The family should be approached – this was the popular feeling expressed by various associations and much of public opinion as well,' explains Houssin.

In July 1994 the French parliament responded to public concern[7] by abandoning the Caillavet Law in favour of new legislation, the Bioethics Law, which tilts the balance back in favour of the family and, in so doing, has seriously undermined the country's opt-out system. 'The idea behind it,' says Houssein, 'is that the human body should be respected and protected, that respect for the human body is related to the dignity of the human person.'

The new law established a national computerized register to allow people who want to opt out to say no. It also forces doctors to approach the families of potential donors, not to ask for the family's consent but to double-check what the dead person's wishes were. In theory France still has an opt-out system; in practice, fears about its corrupting effect on doctors' approach to the dead have so weakened it as to make it unworkable. After the Amiens affair, no doctor is going to risk taking the organs from a potential donor if their family opposes the idea. 'If the family says no, you can't do anything,' says Professor Houssin. 'Presumed consent has been seriously attenuated.'

The Tesnieres, at least, will be pleased at this news: their once generous support of organ transplantation has been fatally undermined by presumed consent. They are now such bitter opponents of spare-part surgery that Alain Tesniere has written the following inscription in his social security card: 'In memory of my son Christophe, I forbid any removal of organs, tissues and other remains from myself and from my son Oliver who is a minor.'

'I'd rather die if I ever needed an organ,' he says. 'I think that a person is unique and that we shouldn't change organs from one person to another. Human beings are not a collection of organs like a car. An organ is part of a person's identity. I prefer to die because I know how doctors practise in France.'

Mireille is just as hostile. 'At the time I thought it was important to help someone to live,' she says. 'But if I had known then everything that I know now I would have lied and told them that Christophe was opposed to organ donation. I think it is inhumane. The doctors took everything they could from Christophe's body and I have to live with that even today.'

The moral quandaries facing Western societies about transplant surgery seem like a luxury when seen from the perspective of a poor nation like India. We agonize about our respect for the dead while they cannot afford to run a widespread public transplant service. India has the medical expertise but it lacks the infrastructure. Its slender resources are fully stretched in providing basic health care to the country's 850 million inhabitants. There are only four cities in the country where transplants are done: Bombay, Delhi, Hyderabad and Madras. If you are lucky, you can have one, but you have to be wealthy. About 80,000 people die there each year for want of a transplant or an artificial kidney. In India, though, the poor have been trying to provide a solution to the donor shortage by selling their organs to the rich. Westerners throw up their hands in horror at the thought of a trade in human organs, and even the Indian government is now doing its best to stamp it out, but organ sales have plenty of respectable supporters. Dr Keschava Chandra Reddy, a kidney specialist at the Lady Willingdon Hospital in Madras, says: 'In a country where you can't even give people clean drinking water to prevent them dying of diarrhoea, malaria, cholera and other easily preventable diseases, you can't expect the Government to lay out

enormous quantities of money to provide a transplant programme. So I think it is foolish and not ethically correct to try and
ban the trade.'

Until recently, it was common to find people outside the Lady
Willingdon Hospital, waiting patiently to register their desire to
sell one of their kidneys. Malathi, a slum-dweller, joined the
queue in 1994 in the hope of buying himself out of the poverty
trap. The going rate for a kidney was 30,000 rupees or £650 – a
small fortune in a country in which most people earn only £25 a
year. Like many poor people in India, Malathi is in debt to a
money-lender. 'It is better to be without a kidney than to be
saddled with a debt,' he explains. 'I couldn't resist the debt
collectors any longer.'

Yet Malathi's presence in the kidney-donor queue was unusual:
most people who decide to sell a kidney in India are women
because traditionally their health has been regarded as less
important than the men's. But, whatever your sex, the dream of
a debt-free life comes true only if you pass a series of tests
designed to weed out unsuitable donors.

'The donor must come with his next-of-kin and some kind of
identification,' says Reddy. 'They have a preliminary chat with a
social worker. Once that person is satisfied, they have a basic
medical test to make sure they are all right. If they pass, a doctor
uses charts to explain where the kidney is situated, what its
functions are, what happens when you remove it and that losing
one is not in the long-term deleterious to their health. I speak to
every single donor and their next-of-kin and I even tell them
there is a small risk to life. Once they are quite sure about it, I ask
them what they plan to do with their money.'

Saraswarthy, a woman in her late thirties and the mother of
two children, passed all the tests and sold one of her kidneys. Half
the money she received went to pay off her husband's debts in the
hope that he would leave his mistress and return home – he did
not – but 10,000 rupees went into a bank account, and a further
5,000 were spent on jewellery for her daughter to use as a dowry
when she marries. She knows quite a lot about kidneys and blood
groups now, although before her operation she had to be told

where her kidneys were and how many she had. 'It wasn't difficult to do,' she says. 'I myself went to the hospital, spoke to the sister and asked to donate a kidney. After my operation ten people came and asked me how to donate a kidney so I took them all along to the hospital. They wanted people with the O blood group so they only took four of them.'

For the past decade, India has turned a blind eye to a trade that the rest of us abhor, because it saves lives. Dr Reddy is a thoughtful man with a bedside manner that would put the most anxious of patients at ease. He asks critics not to bring armchair morality to bear on a nation whose problems they do not understand. 'In this country you get a poor man who goes down into the drains, in the sewage, wearing nothing but a simple loincloth,' he says. 'What he is doing is far more hazardous to himself than donating a kidney for money. But would anybody stop him? Because if they did, who's going to clean the sewage for you? Nobody ever says you're exploiting this poor man because he has to work and he's willing to do it. So I think we have to be very clear in our minds who it is who's being exploited. After all, the person who is buying the kidney is not doing it because he wants to have steak and kidney for lunch! He is doing it to save his life. And the poor guy who's giving it, whatever his reasons may be, is doing it for a beneficial purpose, for himself or for his family. What's wrong with that?'

Such arguments have found little favour among the nation's legislators. Under pressure from international opinion, the central government introduced a law last year banning kidney sales throughout the country.[8] It has already been ratified by several of India's 25 state parliaments, where the only live donations now permitted are between blood relatives. Supporters of the law believe it will force the Government to introduce a proper transplantation service. 'You need quite a lot of public pressure generated in the media,' explains one of the new law's backers, Dr M.A. Mutthusethupathi, the head of the nephrology department at Madras Government Hospital. 'As long as the rich can buy kidneys from poor people, this is a great disincentive to the development of a cadaver (dead body) organ programme. The best means of benefiting the most people in this country is by the adoption of such a programme – and this is being hampered by unregulated organ buying.'

However, the ban on kidney sales has many opponents. Dr Reddy scoffs at the idea that it will result in a public transplant programme. While the law might leave doctors with clear consciences, he thinks it will also leave them with dying patients. 'It's quite ridiculous,' says Reddy, 'because the Government just does not have the money to provide a service of that nature. Such a programme could only affect a minuscule proportion of the population. It certainly will not meet the needs of affected people in any substantial way. We don't have the mechanics; we don't have the infrastructure; we don't have the logistics. Let's get down to brass tacks: assuming a brain-dead road-accident victim is brought to a hospital and the next-of-kin give you permission to take his organs. Somebody has to pay for this. So who is going to pay for the retrieval of the organs? Who is going to pay for the preservation of the organs? Who is going to pay for all the money that's been spent while he was in the Intensive Care Unit? Who's going to pay? And then, once you've got the organs, who are you going to give them to? You're only going to give them to those patients who happen to be on dialysis. And who are those patients? They're the patients who can afford to pay!'

The sale of kidneys has been above board for the past two decades, but Reddy fears that far from ending the trade in organs, a ban will drive it underground. Desperate patients will take desperate measures, whatever the law says, and the only people to benefit will be the unscrupulous. 'No patient who is condemned to death is going to lie back in his bed and say: "So be it. I am going to die!" If that person were your brother, your sister, your son, father or mother, you are going to try and help to save their life. And if that means breaking the law, then so be it. They will try to do this through the underworld. They will get people to pose as relatives. They'll get false matching certificates, false names and it will go on merrily. Only now the patient will have to pay that much more for these services.'

Worse even than the thought of black-market transplants is the fear that a ban on kidney sales will provoke a spate of organ thefts: poor men and women being duped into having a kidney removed to save the lives of rich patients. The English-language press in India periodically highlights stories of abuse that might have been taken from a good crime novel. The victims are always uneducated and unaware of the most basic medical information. The culprits are middle men who deliver unsuspecting individuals into the hands of corrupt doctors and surgeons who remove a kidney without its owner's permission.

One of the most recent of these stories came to light in January 1995 when a labourer turned up at a police station in Bangalore complaining that he had been robbed of an organ. His name is Velu and he comes from the village of Pallipalayam in the neighbouring state of Tamil Nadu. Velu told the police he was earning 25 rupees a day (£0.55) when he was approached by two labour agents called Mohammed Yousuf and Mohammed Hanif, who promised him a job in the city that could earn him four times as much. Velu decided to try his luck, but arrived in Bangalore in August 1994 to find he couldn't get any work. The two agents suggested another way for him to earn a living: that he sell blood to a hospital, and took him to Yelamma Desappa Hospital several times for this purpose. On one of his visits Velu says he became dizzy and lost consciousness. 'I saw the mark [the scar] on my stomach only after I regained consciousness,' he explains. 'I found I had been operated upon. I was stunned. Dr Siddaraju saw me and held my hand and said I would be all right. He said I had had a fall and there was nothing to worry about.'

Dr K. S. Siddaraju is the doctor in charge of the nephrology department at a government-run hospital in Bangalore. But he also works as a consultant at the private Yelamma Desappa hospital. According to Velu, Siddaraju told him he lost his balance after giving blood and had fallen out of a first-floor window. He injured the side of his body and was operated on by two surgeons at the hospital, Dr Dilip Patil and Dr Dilip Dhanpal. Velu was discharged about a week later, and says he was given 5,000 rupees by the doctors and told to go home and rest. 'I used to get tired very quickly,' he explains. 'I could not even lift a

bucket of water. My wife used to say: "Go and see a doctor." But I
didn't. Two or three months later, I had a fight with my brother
who punched me in the stomach. I was in unbearable pain and
did go to a doctor who, on seeing the mark, told me that my
kidney had been removed.'

Velu says he was mystified. He thought he had been operated
on purely to repair the injury that resulted from his fall and that
he had been given the 5,000 rupees in compensation for the
accident. He was so disturbed to find out that he had been
deceived that he went back to Bangalore to find the men who had
taken his kidney. He spoke to Dr Syed Adil Ahmed, the doctor
whom he'd met during his first visits to the hospital. 'I told the
doctor he had removed my kidney under the pretext of taking
blood,' he says. 'He said he had paid me 5,000 rupees and told me
I could not do anything to them. I told them it was wrong on
their part to remove my kidney without my knowledge and asked
for compensation. They were very casual and did not express any
regrets. In fact, I told them I would not pursue the matter if they
gave me some compensation to help me take care of my family.
They did not bother.'

Velu also went to see Dr Siddaraju and claims that he was just
as curt. 'He said I had already been paid 5,000 rupees and asked
me to go back home,' says Velu. ' "Do what you want," he said.'

Velu went to the police – accompanied by six other villagers,
with scars on their sides, who also claimed to have had a kidney
removed without their permission by Siddaraju and his two
medical colleagues. He spoke to Inspector Vincent D'Souza who
believed Velu's story. He was convinced that the three doctors
and the two labour agents were involved in a racket to steal
organs from naïve villagers and he sent a squad of officers to
arrest Dr Siddaraju. 'Dr Siddaraju is the main architect of the
whole episode,' explains D'Souza. 'We have come to know this
during the course of our investigation because the nephrologist
has to decide whether the person is fit for transplantation,
whether the kidney is fit to be transplanted and whether it will
match. It was he who had to decide all that.'

Siddaraju is not a typical crook. He is a neat, polite and

respectful man, who lives in a middle-class district on the outskirts of Bangalore. If he is wealthy, it doesn't show. He drives an old car; he dresses casually; his house is certainly not luxurious – it even lacks air conditioning. So if he is robbing poor people's kidneys to make large sums of money, he doesn't seem to be making a very good job of it. The police thought otherwise. They turned up outside his home in force in the middle of the night and, Siddaraju claims, treated him with scant respect.

'Suddenly I saw some police officers knocking at my door,' he recalls. 'I presumed they had come on behalf of a police officer on whom we had operated just four or five days back. I thought that perhaps something had gone wrong and, in panic, they'd rushed to my residence. So I opened the door and offered them a seat. They only asked me one question: "Are you, Siddaraju, doing organ transplants?" I said yes. All they said was: "Come. We have a case against you." I tried to ring up some friends to tell them that something is going on, but they snapped the telephone wire and bundled me into a jeep . . . I was whisked away at eleven o'clock at night without them even telling my family where I was being taken or what offence I had committed. They thought I had been kidnapped. They didn't think this was a real police action because even the police officer who lives next door said that no policeman would act like this.'

Siddaraju was driven off in his night-shirt and slippers to Frazer police station and says he spent twenty-four hours in a cell before anyone told him that he faced an array of charges, including stealing organs, causing grievous harm by having intoxicants, fabricating false documents, criminal conspiracy, tampering with evidence and wrongful confinement. Inspector D'Souza had already had the two agents and two of the other doctors arrested. His Commissioner of Police then promptly held a press conference. With representatives of the national and international media corps present, the police announced that they'd broken a major organ-theft ring. Once the story hit the headlines, eighty other villagers arrived at the police station, complaining that their kidneys had also been stolen by the same medical team. Inspector D'Souza thought he had a big case on his hands. 'We have referred all these cases to a government expert in transplantation and he has given us an opinion in writing that the doctors have erred,' he says. 'As the investigating officer, I am personally satisfied that we have enough evidence to show that these people are involved in this crime. We are prosecuting them and their case is now pending.'

But is the case as clear-cut as the police would like to believe? Velu has told more than one version of the events leading to the removal of his kidney. He told our film crew that the doctor had said he had fallen from a first-floor window. We checked and found that all the windows on this floor are barred. He told our researcher that he became dizzy and lost consciousness after being given an injection, not after giving blood. And he told his own lawyer that the doctors told him they had operated to take more blood. What is more, a number of other people in and around Velu's home village had sold kidneys before he had his operation. They would have had scars in exactly the same place as Velu, so it seems unlikely that three months would pass before he became suspicious about the scar on his body. There are also questions to be asked about the statements made by some of the other complainants. Shantappa Devirappa, for example, told the police that he had consulted Dr Siddaraju about an ulcer that had been operated on and was causing trouble, and was told that he needed another operation, which he had had at Yelamma Desappa Hospital. Later he accused the doctors of stealing his kidney.

Dr Siddaraju is quick to point out what he thinks is the flaw in this story. 'I am a nephrologist, an expert in renal diseases,' he says. 'I don't see patients with ulcers at all. They go to a gastroenterologist. So this is something which he tried to make up. I don't think there's any truth in his allegations . . . I did see him, but he came to me with the sole intention of donating a kidney and he donated it with his full knowledge and consent.'

Siddaraju protests his innocence – and that of his medical colleagues – of all the charges they face. Under close questioning the doctor appears calm, clear-headed and disturbed by what he sees as the uncritical credibility that the police have given to the statements of Velu and the other complainants. But he didn't do himself any favours when he vanished the moment he was allowed out on bail, giving the distinct impression of a guilty man on the run. That, at least, is how it appeared in the papers. Siddaraju says it wasn't quite like this. 'I was afraid of the police,' he explains. 'I think practically everybody is afraid of the police in our country . . . Because of the treatment that I received on the first day, I knew they were very keen to harass me and that it was going to be repeated in a much more severe form. Knowing the attitude of the police, I felt that I should not be available to them. I did not run away.'

Be that as it may, the police claim that Siddaraju and his colleagues failed to get Velu's informed consent before removing his kidney. They also allege that he did not carry out the most basic of medical investigations – an angiogram and a cross-match test – before the operation. They say that this has been confirmed by an independent transplant specialist. For his part, Siddaraju insists that Velu willingly agreed to the removal of the kidney and that the only money he, Velu, received came from the patient who bought it. He says that all the relevant tests were performed because it is technically impossible to do a transplant without them. There are, says Siddaraju, full records to prove this. 'The angiogram reveals the status of the kidney's blood vessels,' he says, 'the renal artery and renal vein, which we are going to attach to the recipient. The cross-match test tells us whether the kidney will be accepted by the patient or not. Without that knowledge, no surgeon who knows about transplantation will operate . . . I'm really amazed that a medical man who is supposed to know about transplants can make such allegations. Really, this just cannot happen anywhere in the world.'

Siddaraju has been suspended from his job until the court case is over; it could be more than a year before the matter is settled. Despite his predicament, the doctor is charitable towards his accusers. His anger is reserved for the police who, he feels, have succumbed to a growing hysteria about the trade in organs. 'I feel that the complainants are innocent,' he says. 'Their main aim was to get a little extra money. But the police overreacted. They thought that there was something huge and unethical going on

... The police went into action without verifying whether such a thing is possible or not. . . . All the accusations against me are one hundred per cent false . . . I feel that this whole thing is a cooked-up, concocted story.'

Bangalore City Sessions Court must now decide whether Siddaraju and his colleagues are the instigators of an underhand conspiracy or the innocent victims of a deception born of grinding poverty. Whatever the outcome of this case, the ban on kidney sales in a country with no public transplantation service seems bound to lead to serious abuses. The law of supply and demand is straightforward: where there is a shortage of a valuable commodity, someone will find a way to fill the gap – at a price. And India is not the only poor country that has repeatedly thrown up stories of gross exploitation.

In Argentina reporters investigated the disappearance of fourteen-year-old Marcelo Ortiz, a disabled boy living at the Montes de Oca psychiatric hospital near Buenos Aires. His body was later found in the hospital grounds – minus his eyeballs. According to the reports, they had been removed by an employee, who had torn them out with a teaspoon so that his corneas might be sold for transplantation. A judge then revealed a gruesome trade in human organs. Marcelo, he found, was one of more than a thousand patients who had disappeared from the hospital. They were murdered, according to patients still there – killed by poisoning before their eyes were extracted and sold. Some bodies were found in a swamp; others in a sewer. Some had been unceremoniously buried in the local cemetery.

In Russia, Yury Petrovich Dubyagin, a police colonel who works in Moscow city morgue identifying bodies, says that the Mafia is kidnapping children and adults and using their organs for transplants. He has seen scores of corpses with mysterious surgical incisions in their sides. He claims that organ transplantation is one of the most profitable businesses in Russia. There have been many other reports of organ thefts, in Brazil, Colombia, Mexico, Peru and Nepal. Conclusive proof is difficult to obtain so it is hard to ascertain the strength of allegations which have, unfortunately, attracted much sensationalist reporting. But the accumulating evidence is now being taken seriously by international aid organizations. A recent UN report concluded that 'there is . . . mounting evidence of a market for children's organs'.

The subject is increasingly becoming a political hot potato. The American government's Information Agency, for example, has become so worried about the reports – particularly those that implicate rich Americans – that it has given Todd Leventhal, the agency's programme officer for countering disinformation and misinformation, the task of pouring cold water on the issue. He dismisses organ theft as an 'urban legend'. While most concerned organizations want to prevent such gross abuses, Leventhal is maintaining that they do not exist. 'In the eight years in which these allegations have circulated no one has ever produced any credible evidence to support them,' he told a meeting of the European Society for Organ Transplantation in October 1995.[9]

Whether Mr Leventhal is the best person to distinguish between myth and reality is open to question. During the Cold War he was a US government propaganda chief, charged with countering what he calls disinformation from the Soviet Union. Now he is waging an effective campaign against another enemy: the theft of organs from unsuspecting victims. Leventhal is discrediting such reports – because bad news stories tend to depress organ-donation rates and have, he claims, led to attacks on Americans. But there have been so many reports of organ theft that it is hard to credit there can be so much smoke without at least a few small fires, and it seems likely that these will continue to smoulder as long as there is a shortage of transplantable organs.

7

A Pig to Save Your Bacon

In August 1992 David White, the Cambridge immunologist, spent four days in Paris at a meeting of the International Transplantation Society. The visit was no secret. While he was away, the local press ran a story about his trip, so it was common knowledge that he was not at home. It was late at night when he returned, unlocked his front door, dumped his travel bag in the hallway and switched on the lights. The sight that greeted his tired eyes shocked him to the core. 'I walked in and the whole house looked like a bomb had hit it,' he says. 'There was tomato ketchup all over the ceiling. They had pulled all the books out of my bookcases and got a six-pack of beer and poured it all over the books. They took bleach and wrote "murderer" on the carpets.'

The damage was the work of militant animal rights activists. It was a blunt warning to White to abandon work that he believes will provide a solution to the shortage of organ donors. Three months later they vandalized his home again. White installed a burglar alarm, but even that did not keep his attackers at bay. In 1993, his housekeeper heard a noise at the front door. 'They'd poured petrol through the cat-flap,' he says. 'She went to the door, smelt the petrol and pressed the panic button on the alarm and they ran away without setting fire to the house. They came back again about a year ago, took a garden hose and forced open a skylight, which didn't set off the alarm, stuck the hose through the window, turned it on and left it running. It flooded the whole of the ground floor and eventually set off the alarm. The carpets were ruined and, worst of all, the parquet flooring. You should see my insurance bill now.'

The police have still not caught the perpetrators of these attacks. David White is the focus of such anger because he is trying to solve the donor shortage by putting animal organs into humans. To do so, he is working at the cutting edge of transplant immunology in genetically engineering pigs for a company called Imutran in Cambridge so that their organs will be accepted by the human body. His work could produce an unlimited supply of transplant organs and an end to the lottery of the waiting list. It could also make a fortune for Sandoz, the company that makes Cyclosporin and that is now providing some of the money for the project. Sandoz has been quick to realize the windfall that transplantable animal organs could bring. Forty thousand or so transplants took place world-wide in 1994. With an unlimited supply of organs, this could grow to four hundred thousand. But this work is highly controversial and some people fear that such a high-tech solution could be unethical, impractical and potentially dangerous. 'We don't believe that it is morally right to genetically engineer animals for spare parts for human organs,' complains Malcolm Eames of the Genetics Forum, a pressure group that campaigns for the democratic control of biotechnology. 'The central issue is that it is wrong to take a life to save a life. As far as medical technical advances go, we should be attempting to move away from the use of animals for medicine.'

Such sentiments are fine in theory, but surgeons faced with dying patients have hard choices to make and many would say that when there is no alternative treatment it is morally justified to sacrifice an animal's life to save a human being. After all, there would be *no* transplant surgery but for the thousands of dogs, cats, mice and rats that have died in experimental laboratories and only the most diehard of anti-vivisectionists would suggest abandoning transplantation in atonement for these past sins.

The use of animal organs themselves is quite another matter: the history of transplant surgery is dotted with attempts to save patients' lives with a 'xenograft', the technical term for the transplant of an organ from one species of animal into another. The scientific and ethical problems were daunting and many who stepped into this controversial arena paid a high price for their efforts: nearly all their patients died rapid deaths; the surgeons' reputations nose-dived and one even faced death threats.

The earliest attempts had been made in France and Germany at the turn of the century, and used kidneys taken from a pig, a goat and a Macaque monkey. They failed.[1] More than half a century passed before anyone had the courage to try again. By then, a much clearer understanding had been reached of the problems of such cross-species transplants: it was known, for example, that organs grafted between such distantly related species as humans and the pig or the goat would be subjected to hyperacute rejection, which could not be controlled by drugs. Yet that did not apply to xenografts between closely related species: it was believed that the human body would react to an organ from, say, a chimpanzee or a baboon, much as it would to an organ transplanted from another person. Rejection should be controllable by normal drug therapy. In the early 1960s, as kidney transplantation took off, surgeons first became aware of the desperate shortage of transplantable organs. 'The number of living donors was limited and renal dialysis programmes as an option were few in number,' says the liver transplant surgeon Tom Starzl. 'Desperate potential kidney recipients were piling up faster than places could be found for them.'[2]

It was logical, therefore, to wonder if the organs of our nearest relatives in the animal kingdom – chimpanzees and baboons, for example – could be used to solve the donor shortage and save human lives. However, the killing of animals with many characteristics in common with human beings was highly emotive, and the surgeons who first used these animals conducted their work in secret. In November 1963 Keith Reemtsma, a surgeon at the Tulane University School of Medicine in America, bought an 80-pound chimpanzee called Adam that had been rejected by a circus for bad temper and poor behaviour. Reemtsma wanted to graft the animal's kidneys into forty-three-year-old Jefferson Davis, a dock worker dying of kidney failure. 'It was obviously very controversial,' he recalls, 'because there were those who thought that this was too highly experimental. Since we had such difficulties in human transplants, [they thought], why would anyone take the additional step of going from non-human to human?'

Reemtsma had answers for his critics. He pointed out the difficulty he had in finding transplantable human kidneys: the idea of removing them from dead bodies was still new in 1963 and, so far, had not been consistently successful. He also said that the blood groups and genetic make-up of chimpanzees and humans were so similar that such a cross-species transplant should stand a good chance of surviving. His assistant surgeon Prentiss Smith did not share his confidence. 'Keith,' he joked with his boss, who was born on an Indian reservation, 'if this doesn't work you can always go back to the Navajo reservation and straighten out the hymnals and pass the collection plate.'[3]

Reemtsma wasn't put off. He discussed the ethics of the new procedure with his colleagues. He talked about it at length with the patient, agreeing only to use the chimpanzee's kidney if no suitable human donor became available. Eventually he transplanted both the chimpanzee's kidneys into Jefferson Davis. The press wasn't told about the operation, a decision that Reemtsma defends by saying that his patient's right to privacy overrode the public's right to know. It is clear, though, that he wanted to avoid a public row. The sacrifice of a chimpanzee – even one that had anyway outlived its useful life and was going to be destroyed – would have raised the hackles of animal lovers. It was only when it seemed that the transplant was going to work that the surgeon stuck his head above the parapet.

Six weeks after his operation, an apparently healthy Jefferson Davis was wheeled into a press conference. 'I feel better now than I have in five years,' he told the assembled journalists. 'I was worried, of course, but not about the animal business. I knew it would be a monkey. It didn't bother me. All I wanted to do was survive. I feel wonderful.'[4]

Davis's good health didn't last. Three weeks after the news conference and nine weeks after the transplant, he died of pneumonia because the drugs he was taking to prevent rejection had weakened his resistance to infection. Reemtsma didn't head back to the Navajo Reservation, though. He tried again – five times altogether in the next three months.[5] His best effort involved a dying schoolteacher whom he kept alive for nine months with chimpanzee kidneys transplanted in January 1964. The rest of the patients died within a few weeks of their operations.

'We would emphasize . . . that we regard this work as wholly experimental,' Reemtsma reported in 1964. 'Under the circumstances only the most stringent precautions will make such work justified and justifiable.'[6] Secrecy was one such precaution and Keith Reemtsma was not the only surgeon to duck controversy by avoiding the glare of publicity. While he was in the middle of the series of chimpanzee transplants, Claude Hitchcock, of the Hennepin County Hospital in Minneapolis, revealed that he had transplanted a baboon's kidney into a sixty-five-year-old woman in February 1963, nine months before Reemtsma had started. Fearing a public row, Hitchcock did not tell the outside world about this operation until it became clear that Reemtsma was having more success with his chimpanzee kidneys. The reason for this coy approach was clear: the baboon's organ had worked for only four days before its main artery clotted and the transplant failed.[7]

The next sacrifice of a chimpanzee for its organs caused such a row in the medical world that it cast a pall over xenotransplantation. James Hardy, an American cardiac surgeon, used its heart to try to save a patient's life in 1964 – three years before the first human-heart transplant, when the idea of replacing a human heart raised as many ethical questions as did the killing of a chimpanzee. Hardy misjudged the mood of America: the country was not ready to give its surgeons *carte blanche* to experiment in two such contentious areas at once. Moral and professional indignation were his only rewards.

For several years Hardy had been transplanting hearts and lungs between dogs in the experimental laboratories of the University of Mississippi Medical Centre in Jackson. Most of his transplanted animals died within a month of their operations, although a handful survived, including one dog that lived for more than a year. However, Hardy felt ready to try to save a patient's life with the new technique. He wanted to use a human heart but faced two quandaries. He considered the technique still too experimental to use on someone with any real life expectancy because failure might shorten their life, so he would only perform a transplant on a patient who was near death. But to operate on someone whose body was already very weak meant that their chance of survival was limited. Hardy also could not take a beating heart out of a brain-dead person. This would have been unthinkable at that time – the human heart was still treated with too much reverence in 1964. But he knew that allowing the donor heart to stop naturally would damage it and reduce his chances of success. Hardy resolved this predicament by deciding to transplant a human heart only if, by chance, the donor and recipient were in the hospital on the verge of death at precisely the same moment. He would wait for the donor heart to stop beating, then, with the relatives' permission, start it again while he opened the chest and prepare to remove it. The chances of these circumstances occurring together in the small university hospital were remote, and Hardy thought it might be months or even years before the opportunity arose. He devised a back-up plan after visiting Keith Reemtsma in New York, where he had been impressed by the results of Reemtsma's six chimpanzee xenografts. Hardy bought two chimpanzees which he housed in the university's experimental laboratories. If he was unable to find a human heart he would use a heart from one of the animals in a dying patient.

He didn't have to wait long. In January 1964, Boyd Rush, a sixty-eight-year-old retired upholsterer, suffered a heart-attack in the caravan in which he lived alone in Laurel Trailer Park near Jackson in Mississippi. He had lain unconscious until a neighbour found him. 'He must have been there two days and nights on the floor,' explains his sister Mrs J.H. Thompson. 'This neighbour called an ambulance. The doctor does not know if he ever knew anything that was going on or not . . . He had so many blood clots in his face and one foot was black.'[8]

Rush was at death's door by the time he reached the university hospital. His pulse was irregular. He was in a coma. His damaged heart was so weak that it was no longer able to pump enough blood round his body, as a result of which the lower part of his left leg was gangrenous. Boyd Rush was not expected to live more than a few hours. Hardy decided to operate in a last-ditch effort to save his patient's life. He would amputate the gangrenous leg and remove any further blood clots in the heart. But the patient's chances were slim and, as chance would have it, there was a suitable human heart donor in the hospital, a brain-damaged patient being kept alive by a ventilator, who looked as if he might die at just the right moment. If Rush's heart stopped during the operation, Hardy decided he would give him a new one. The relatives of the donor and the recipient both gave permission for a transplant to take place.[9] Time was now of the essence.

'We rushed the patient into the operating room when his blood pressure fell to sixty,' recalls James Hardy. 'It was obvious that if any transplant was going to be done it had to be done right then and there . . . but just as we were getting the patient on the heart-lung machine his heart stopped any effective beat. So here we were: we had the patient held alive on the heart-lung machine and what do we do because the possible human donor hadn't died? He was not at the point where we could take his heart.'

If Hardy switched off the heart-lung machine, Boyd Rush would die within minutes. His only chance of life now was the healthy heart beating inside the largest of the two chimpanzees that Hardy had bought for just such an eventuality. The surgeon was aware of the controversy that might follow a decision to use the animal's heart and decided to let a show of hands decide whether Boyd Rush should receive the animal's heart.

'The people who were at the operating table had to be polled,' Hardy explains. 'I said: "This is a hazardous situation publicity-wise and, in many people's minds, morally, so I don't want any recriminations later on from this team. We will get plenty from elsewhere." So I said: "What do you say?" And they all agreed but one and he said: "Well, I'm not going to vote against it but I'm not going to vote for it either." He may have been the wisest, but the four of us there at the operating table agreed to go ahead with the chimpanzee transplantation.'

The chimpanzee was tranquillized and brought into an operating theatre next door to the one in which Boyd Rush now lay, his diseased heart exposed in the centre of his open chest. An hour after Rush's life-blood had been re-routed through the heart-lung machine, his new heart was in place. It was 9 p.m.

when James Hardy placed the metal paddles of the defibrillator on either side of the chimpanzee's heart and shocked it into life.

'I had little doubt that the heart could be put in,' he says. 'The technique's exactly the same in the animal as it is in the human being. But we didn't know whether it would start beating in the human being. It was just unknown . . . I can tell you that when I saw that heart begin to beat – with a forceful beat – it was a huge relief, because at one time we were looking at an empty chest . . . I said: "At least we're in business. At least we're going to have a heart that's going to do something for a while." '

But it didn't beat for very long. The chimp's heart was not large enough to support Boyd Rush, given the patient's poor condition. Hardy attached a pacemaker, and even massaged it by hand, but after two hours Boyd Rush was allowed to die. His death gave birth to intense controversy. The hospital authorities did their best to play down the affair; they had already tried to restrict entry to the operating theatre by stationing a security guard outside the doors, but twenty-five people cajoled their way in. The transplant team were forbidden to speak to the press but as it was clear that the news would leak out, the hospital's director of public information prepared a short statement which 'omitted' to mention that a chimpanzee's heart had been used in the transplant. A few days later, rumour had it that Boyd Rush's donor had been a living human. The hospital authorities had to admit the truth and the press pack descended in force on the University of Mississippi Medical Centre.

'There was a tremendous commotion following his transplant,' says Hardy. 'Anytime you do something of that nature that hasn't been done before you take a risk, there's no two ways about it. On the other hand, if you're going to be an investigator, then sooner or later you've got to get into the patient arena. You've got to move out of the laboratory and into the hospital and use it for some appropriate purpose.'

Many people, however, professional colleagues included, did not think the use of a chimpanzee heart appropriate. A few days later Hardy was invited to give a talk on heart transplantation at the Sixth International Transplantation Conference in the elegant surroundings of New York City's Waldorf Astoria Hotel. The moderator of the meeting was Dr Wilhelm Kolff, who had invented the artificial kidney machine. 'Kolff called my name to speak next,' Hardy recalls, 'but before I was allowed to begin he said to the large audience: "In Mississippi they keep the chimpanzees in one cage and the Negroes in another cage, don't they, Dr Hardy?" '

Hardy was stunned. In 1964 America was in a ferment over civil rights. There were angry protests from black people demanding an end to racism and inequality, while the Ku Klux Klan were at the height of a violent racist campaign and the FBI was under fire for failing to investigate racially motivated murders. Kolff later told Hardy that he had been joking[10] – but his words and their effect on the audience are burnt into Hardy's memory. 'This introduced . . . the huge problem of the bitter integration struggle currently raging in Mississippi along with the use of a lower primate heart for transplantation,' he says. 'I frankly admit that, for one of the few times in my professional career, I was taken aback and did poorly. The audience was palpably hostile . . . I gave our experience as it happened but there was not a single hand of applause thereafter. It was a dismal day.'[11]

Hardy never transplanted another animal organ. He says he wanted someone else to take the heat. 'The aftermath of the first heart transplant was a searing experience for me,' he says. 'It was the first time my clinical integrity had ever been challenged. . . . It hardened me for ever.'[12]

After Hardy, chimpanzees were given a wide berth by most transplant surgeons.[13] Our closest relative in the animal kingdom might have been the surgeons' logical first choice, but chimps were too close to humans for the comfort of the rest of society. Ethics, not genetics, won the argument.

For the transplant surgeon, the next best thing to the chimpanzee was the baboon, another close relative of humans with organs that, when grafted, should not be destroyed by hyperacute rejection. The baboon was not an endangered species and surgeons hoped the use of its organs would not provoke emotive protests. But they were wrong. In 1984, Leonard Bailey, a highly skilled American cardiac surgeon, transplanted a baboon heart into a baby girl and found himself in even deeper water than Hardy. The rewards for his efforts were a police guard, a flak jacket and a barrage of criticism.

Bailey wanted to save the lives of young babies born with incurable heart defects at Loma Linda University Medical Centre, a private hospital an hour's drive east of Los Angeles, run by the Seventh Day Adventist Church[14] and well known for its paediatric heart surgery. Bailey would have preferred to use human hearts for his pioneering surgery but, like Hardy, the shortage of organs forced him to consider using animals. 'It boiled down essentially to baboons,' he says. 'They were readily available . . . and we could study their immune systems and see how compatible they might be with the human immune system. In fact, we found that there's an awful lot of substance shared between ourselves and subhuman primates.'

Since the mid 1970s, Bailey had been perfecting the technique of xenotransplantation in the university's experimental laboratories by grafting new hearts taken from lambs and piglets into young goats. It had not been easy: there had been so little interest in what he was doing that he had had to pass the collecting hat round his colleagues and put in his own money to keep the research going.[15] To add insult to injury, several of the scientific reports he wrote about his animal transplants were rejected by a number of medical journals. But transplantation itself had only developed in the face of considerable opposition from the medical establishment, and Bailey took consolation from the knowledge that not every medical advance wins immediate acceptance in the wider scientific community. Also, some of his transplanted animals had survived for six months with ordinary doses of immuno-suppression – and he had achieved other interesting results: 'We got a huge stream of data,' he explains, 'suggesting that we were really on to something important, that the new-born baby's immune system might be more tolerant in general than a grown-up's immune system and that long-term survival might be possible even though you had your heart transplanted as a new-born.'

Bailey had done no experimental cross-species transplants on monkeys. Despite this, the introduction of Cyclosporin in the early 1980s convinced him that a baboon's heart could save the life of a child and he applied to Loma Linda's ethical committee[16] for permission to do the operation. After what Bailey calls fourteen months of agonizing, in October 1984 he finally got the go-ahead to perform five such operations. The committee agreed that he could transplant baboon hearts into children born with hypoplastic left-heart syndrome. This is a fatal condition affecting one in 12,000 new-born babies in which the main pumping chamber of the heart (the left ventricle) and the main artery leading out of the heart (the aorta), are seriously under-developed. Such children find it difficult to breathe, suffer from extreme fatigue and usually die within two weeks of birth. Two days before Bailey received the permission he sought, a girl with a hypoplastic heart had been born in Barstow, California. The identity of this child has never been revealed, and she is still known only as 'Baby Fae'. She was referred to Loma Linda Medical Centre because of the hospital's good reputation in paediatric heart surgery. Tests revealed that Baby Fae's heart problems were irreparable. Her distressed parents were told that nothing could be done for the child. This was the standard practice with children suffering from such a severe defect at Loma Linda Medical Centre. After the family had left the hospital, the cardiologist in charge of Baby Fae's care asked Bailey if he would be interested in trying to save her life with a baboon heart transplant. Bailey read the case notes and decided to call the parents. It was a fateful decision. Soon her young life would be front-page news all over the world. There would be endless speculation about her health and welfare, and heated debates about the ethics of the operation she was about to undergo.

'We invited the parents to think it over and bring the baby back if they were interested in this form of experimental therapy,' says Bailey. 'They expressed an interest in doing this and we spent the next several days matching the baby's immune system to a panel of baboons and selected one against whom the baby was least responsive.'

Before the tests could be completed, Baby Fae took a sudden

turn for the worse. Her ailing heart could not pump sufficient blood around her frail body and her lungs began to fill with liquid. Bailey put the child on a ventilator, which bought him just enough time to finish the tests and choose the baboon. The baby's life continued to slip away. Both she and Leonard Bailey had reached the point of no return. '[The] baby was dying and was clearly going to die. We'd struggled with her through the night and we felt that, compassionately, we should go ahead and see where it would lead.'

Had Bailey known in advance where he was heading, he might have had second thoughts. At 7.30 a.m. on 26 October, Baby Fae lay anaesthetized in a Loma Lind operating theatre, her body cooled to two-thirds of its normal temperature, her chest opened and a heart-lung machine keeping her alive. In the hospital's animal laboratories Bailey removed the heart of the seven-month-old female baboon. Its blood group didn't match Baby Fae's – but its tissue group did, and Bailey thought this would be more important. The heart was no bigger than a walnut. He placed it in a cold salt solution and carried it up to the operating theatre in which the child's life was held in suspended animation. Four hours after the operation began, the new heart began to beat spontaneously as Bailey relaxed the metal clamps allowing the baby's blood to flow through its chambers.

'There was absolute awe,' recalls Sandra Nehlsen-Cannarella, the immunologist brought in from a New York hospital to choose the most suitable baboon for Baby Fae. 'I don't think there was a dry eye in the room.'

Surgically, the operation was a complete success. Baby Fae was plucked from the point of death and returned to the land of the living, thanks to a baboon heart that showed every sign of being able to support the child's small body. It was an exciting moment in the history of Loma Linda Medical Centre and the transplant team were keen to tell the world of their achievement. Sandra Nehlsen-Cannarella called the operation 'one of the biggest overdue advances in our field'.[17] There was, she said, 'an overwhelming feeling of accomplishment and satisfaction'[18] among the transplant team. Leonard Bailey claimed: 'We know more about new-born heart transplant surgery and immunology than anyone on the globe right now.'[19]

The medical centre was rapidly besieged with reporters hungry for news of the world's youngest heart transplant patient. 'It was the first time that a baby had been transplanted,' says Bailey, 'and the whole world was made aware of it. This was a fairly naïve University in terms of the big world and I don't think anyone here had any notion that so much notice would be taken of this baby. There were hundreds of people – trucks, satellites and that sort of stuff all over the campus. They were here for days. You couldn't turn around.'

Baby Fae did well for the first few days of her new life, but voices of protest soon drowned the voices of triumph. Two days after the operation, militant animal rights' supporters mounted a picket outside the hospital, spearheaded by people who took a fundamentalist view of the use of animals in medical research. The sacrifice of a baboon to save the life of a baby was anathema to their naïve but strictly moral views. They carried placards reading 'Stop the Torture' and 'Ghoulish Tinkering Is Not Science'. They likened Leonard Bailey to Joseph Mengele. They even held a memorial service for the baboon.

'I am opposed to scientific experiments on animals and feel strongly about the invalidity of the science that uses animals,' says Margo Tannenbaum, one of the picket organizers. 'I think it is terribly bad science. Using parts from animals for surgery is completely unnatural. The body is made to reject anything that comes from another animal. The work that Bailey does only ends up retarding and hurting mankind.'

The baboon heart beating inside Baby Fae's chest was becoming the focus of an ethical storm that carried far beyond the intense ranks of the anti-vivisection movement. The hospital authorities reacted to the growing furore by dispatching security guards with dogs to patrol the grounds and to protect the nursery where Baby Fae was recovering from her operation. To make matters worse, Bailey's fellow doctors now broke the normally united ranks of the medical profession to voice strong criticism of the operation.

'There has never been a successful cross-species transplant,' insisted John Najarian, the Minnesota-based transplant surgeon. 'To try it now is merely to prolong the dying process. I think Baby Fae is going to reject her heart.'[20]

Jacques Losman, a cardiac surgeon from the Beth Israel Hospital in Newark, New Jersey, who once worked on Christiaan Barnard's transplant programme in South Africa, said, 'All animal experiments have shown that transplants from one species to another fail – be it between dogs and fox, dogs and wolf or [between] different animals. I don't think there was much scientific basis to believe that this would work.'[21]

The days went by and Baby Fae stayed alive – but the story began to spin out of control. The director of California's Organ Procurement Agency claimed that a human heart had been available at the time Baby Fae was given the baboon heart. Bailey denied this: he said he had not been told about the human heart until two days after he had operated on the child and, anyway, had he waited any longer, she would have died. The question of 'informed consent' was discussed vociferously when it became clear that a few American hospitals were offering a risky corrective operation for infants born with hypoplastic hearts.[22] The press wanted to see the consent form signed by Baby Fae's parents to check that they had been told of this option, but the hospital refused to release the document. And there was a row about the string of factual errors in the hospital's statements to the media. The press tactfully called these 'mis-statements', but some, like Baby Fae's age at the time of the operation, wrongly given as fourteen days, had been lies told deliberately to protect the privacy of the parents.

Bailey's worst headache, though, was caused by the animal rights activists, and particularly by the few protesters so blinded by their convictions that they were ready to threaten acts of violence to defend the welfare of baboons. 'My family suffered immensely,' he says. 'We had to have police live in our home, for instance. Our personal mail was opened by the police department for over a year. I wasn't allowed to appear in public without a bullet-proof vest under my clothing because of the array of threats that came through in those days.'[23]

This was a clash of moral philosophies, with acts of violence justified by appeals to the greater good. For the protesters, all animals have equal moral worth – there is no hierarchy of species with humans at the top – and a few felt justified in using violence against a member of their own species if it succeeded in ending violence against members of another.

'I don't understand why man thinks that he is so far more evolved and his life worth so much more than any other life form on earth,' says Margo Tannenbaum, who was not implicated in any violence.[24] 'How do we know that we are the best of life on this earth and that the goat isn't? How do we know that the goat won't evolve and that we won't totally eradicate ourselves and become an endangered species? I mean, who tells us that we are the only species on the face of the earth that can turn around and use every other species?'

For Leonard Bailey and the transplant team, humans have a higher moral value and so the desire to save the life of a member of our own species is sufficient reason to end the life of a member of another. 'Some say that the animal's life is just as valuable as the human baby's life and that we have no business taking the animal's life,' says Bailey. 'I'm sensitive to that point of view, I have some misgivings about it myself. But as I look at the planet earth and the various species that are scattered about, there is a certain survival of the fittest that goes on in nature, the lion eats the zebra and so forth, and it seems to me, as a human being, that my obligation is to my own species first. If there is a way to support the life of a member of my own species, even though it requires the sensitive and caring taking of a subhuman primate life, I think I'm obligated to pursue that course of action.'

The saving grace for Leonard Bailey in this bitter argument was Baby Fae herself. While she was alive, sustained by the baboon heart beating inside her chest, she was justification of his belief in the morality of his actions. For two weeks Bailey's patient defied all the immunological odds and made a good recovery. Then the inevitable happened. Her body appeared to be rejecting the transplant. Bailey increased the dose of Cyclosporin, but a few days later Baby Fae's kidneys began to fail, followed in quick succession by her heart. The transplant team worked desperately hard to keep her alive: they dialysed her to cleanse her blood; they placed her in an oxygen tent to assist her weakening heart. They even tried cardiac massage. But Baby Fae died on 15 November 1984. Bailey later discovered that rejection hadn't killed Baby Fae. Instead the mis-match between her blood and that of the baboon had caused the child's red blood cells to stick together, blocking her arteries and veins. In fact, the heart was the last organ to fail. It had kept her alive for twenty days, longer than any other patient given an animal's heart, but not long enough to silence Bailey's medical and moral critics.

'She lived just long enough to captivate us into thinking she was going to survive and the world would be a better place as a result,' says Bailey, 'and when she died we were all heartbroken I'm afraid. But she taught us a lot. She was the pioneer, actually, not us.'

Bailey never performed the other four baboon-heart transplants for which he had been given permission by the hospital's ethics committee. Baby Fae's short life had been so traumatic for him that he wanted to spare his family any further ordeals. His growing qualms about using primates for spare-part surgery also played a part in the decision. 'I am not sure that I know where I stand on this,' he says. 'I take a lead from my children. Neither they nor I like the idea of taking the lives of healthy primates and the only way we can justify it is the notion that we can save a member of our own species. . . . It gives you pause for reflection. You have to continually check what you are doing against public opinion, whether or not it is justifiable, whether it is right.'[25]

It was abundantly clear after Baby Fae's death that primate organs were not the answer to the donor shortage. The killing of monkeys to save human lives was too emotive ever to be a practical solution even if, with time and patience, the problem of rejection was overcome. Yet, from an immunological perspective, these organs were the only practical source: those from more distant species – dogs, sheep, pigs, calves, for example – all provoked such a fierce hyperacute rejection that existing immuno-suppressive treatments were impotent. The reaction can be so severe that a pig's heart put into a human will turn black and cease beating in about fifteen minutes.[26]

By the mid 1980s a combination of moral doubts and immunological concerns seemed therefore to have ruled out the use of animal organs to solve the donor shortage. It was also patently obvious that the gap would never be filled by human organs, no matter how much the law was modified or how many appeals made to people's consciences. Many surgeons were resigned to the shortage and all the dilemmas that it implied. One or two, though, had other ideas. John Wallwork, a transplant surgeon at Papworth Hospital in Cambridge, wondered why it was not possible for organs from more distant species to survive in humans. The pig, for example, would be ideal: it's organs are the right size for humans; it is not an endangered species and pigs are sacrificed in their thousands every day for the benefit of humanity's stomachs. 'We already use animal parts for lots of things in medicine,' he says. 'And I don't think there is any big moral dilemma in breeding pigs for food – and if you breed them for food it seems to me much more of a morally defensible stand to breed them to improve people's lives. So I don't think there's an issue there.'

The problem, of course, was hyperacute rejection. But spare-part surgery owed its existence to the convictions of doctors who had refused to be daunted by sceptics and critics, and Wallwork, an irrepressible optimist, continued in the honourable tradition. 'When I first started this, people said, "Oh, you're crazy, this will never happen,"' he says. 'I have an analogy for this: it's a bit like sitting in a London club in the fog in November at the turn of the century having a brandy and some guy comes up to you and says, "Look, within our lifetime we'll be able to get into a tube of steel and fly to New York at twice the speed of sound, drinking champagne." Then you'd go home to your wife and say, "I met this real nutter tonight!" But it happened. And this is going to happen and it's going to change the way we think, not just about transplantation but eventually the way we think about medicine.'

In 1984 Wallwork joined forces with the immunologist, David White, to form a company in Cambridge called Imutran, which aimed, one day, to save human lives with pigs' organs. Hard cash was needed – but Britain's Medical Research Council was only prepared to put up £17,000. Wallwork went to America where he persuaded Warburg Pincus, a New York City bank, to produce enough money to enable White to begin the daunting task of discovering whether there was a way to make Wallwork's dream come true.[27] 'We said, let's find out what it is that makes a pig a pig; a zebra a zebra; a crocodile a crocodile and a man a man,' says Wallwork. 'What is the pigness of pig – and the zebraness of zebra – that stops us being able to transplant them?'

The key to the problem of hyperacute rejection is a toxic protein in the blood called 'complement', released by the body when it senses the presence of an organ from a distant species and which destroys the transplanted organ by punching holes in its cells. Once released, complement will destroy any cells with which it comes into contact, even the cells of the body producing it. White realized that there must, therefore, be some kind of a marker – a 'flag' – on the surface of all our cells that prevents the complement from being released. 'There's obviously some kind of a message system,' he explains, 'that says to the complement: "We're on your side, please don't destroy us. Go and find some unfriendly bacteria to blow up instead." And that message system is a group of proteins that are on every cell in our body.'

There are several complement-blocking proteins, but White believed that three – known as DAF, MCP and CD59 – were the most important. After conducting laboratory tests with mice, he devised a plan for beating hyperacute rejection. He decided to inject the genes responsible for making DAF, MCP and CD59 into a fertilized pig's egg. He hoped that they would be incorporated into the genetic code, appearing on one pair of the animal's chromosomes[28] so that when the piglet was born, its cells would come equipped with a minute 'flag' telling the human complement that it was friend not foe.[29] If an organ from this pig was then transplanted into a human, White believed that the complement would be fooled into thinking it had come from a person and so wouldn't destroy it. Instead of altering the human body to prevent it attacking the transplant, he was going to alter the genetic structure of the organ to prevent hyperacute rejection.

'I like to think that what we are doing is making non-stick frying pans,' says White, who has the knack of explaining complicated scientific concepts with easy-to-understand analogies. 'We are putting Teflon on the organs that we want to transplant and it's the Teflon – the 'flags' – that will protect them. The more the protection, the less likely they are to be rejected. So we look for the heart or the lungs with the most Teflon on.'

If White succeeded, he would usher in a golden era of transplantation: there would be an end to waiting lists and patients dying needlessly for want of suitable organs. Yet it was an immense scientific challenge: it meant genetically engineering the pig to ensure that the human 'flag' was present on all the cells in its body. It was also highly controversial, as White soon discovered when animal rights activists smashed up his home and threatened his life.

The violence, though, did not end Imutran's work. After little more than a decade, Wallwork and White's vision is taking shape in the East Anglian countryside where a herd of 300 to 400 genetically engineered pigs are housed. These are second-generation animals; the first generation was born in 1992 from fertilized eggs to which White had added the gene that produces DAF.[30] Because of the laws governing inheritance, these animals only had the gene on one half of the relevant pair of chromosomes on which it appeared. To maximize his chances of preventing hyperacute rejection, White cross-bred these animals, producing a second generation in 1995 that had the gene on both halves of the pair. Only a handful of people know exactly where the pigs are kept, secrecy that's essential, White insists, because some animal rights activists would like nothing better than to wreak havoc at the hermetically sealed, clinically controlled pig-sty.

'We restrict access to this facility a great deal,' he explains, standing in a large pen surrounded by his squealing swine, which look indistinguishable from their unaltered cousins. 'It's not because we're ashamed of anything that goes on here – or because we do anything secret. We're very proud of the way we look after our pigs. We're very open about what we do and how we do it.

But the real problem is, we don't want a band of nutters coming across the fields and releasing transgenic pigs all over the Cambridge countryside. I think it's a great shame that we have to take these enormous security measures. But frankly they've been forced upon us.'

The motivation behind White and Wallwork's work might be well intentioned, but genetic engineering raises serious ethical and practical concerns. Many thoughtful people object in principle to any experimental use of animals – let alone altering their genetic structure and then killing them for their organs. The critics of this high-tech solution to the donor shortage believe that the doctors backing the plan are dragging our moral values down a path that we have spent most of this century travelling up. 'We should be attempting to move away from the use of animals for medicine,' says Malcolm Eames of the Genetics Forum. 'We see in our society a growing respect and compassion for these animals and we should be attempting to exploit technology in a way which allows us to lessen our dependence on animals. There is a range of practical administrative measures which could provide a solution to the organ shortage. The thing is that none of these measures offers potential profits for commercial companies to invest in – unlike transgenic animals. We need to take a broader perspective in improving human health rather than developing bizarre new techniques.'

Such words find little favour with White and Wallwork. They disagree on all the fundamental points. There are no real alternatives to the donor shortage, they feel. There will always be a shortage of human organs. As for the moral issues, pigs are domesticated animals bred to provide food for humans. If you can eat a ham sandwich, you can use pigs for experimental research designed to save human lives – provided, of course, that it is conducted humanely.

'I'm personally very fond of animals,' says White. 'I mean I can't even bring myself to kill the mole that's digging up my grass. I think there are limits to the exploitation of animals – different cultures have different limits. For example, I find bull fighting objectionable. But I'm very comfortable with the way we use animals experimentally. Many people may not appreciate the stringency of the laws controlling animal experimentation in this country. The Home Office has a network of inspectors, medically or veterinary qualified individuals, who literally come into the operating theatre when we're doing transplants, watch us doing it, make sure that we give the animals analgesia so that they feel no pain.'

However, the use of organs from genetically engineered animals raises practical questions that demand serious consideration. How do we know, for example, that they will not inadvertently give the recipient an illness suffered by the animal? Not so long ago health officials were thrown into panic by the prospect of humans contracting bovine spongiform encephalopathy (BSE, a disease of cattle), after eating beef. So the possibility of a person being infected by a bacterium or virus from the pig's heart beating in their chest is not far-fetched.

'The highest risk is undoubtedly when you put a human heart into a human chest because, of course, human diseases are ubiquitous,' says White. 'As you go down through the species there are fewer and fewer diseases that can infect humans. But there are some, and we have instituted a large research programme screening our pigs to make quite sure that none of the diseases – or even potential diseases – that a pig could give to a person are contained in these animals. So you are going to be looking at the healthiest pigs anywhere in the world.'

Animal rights activists pour cold water on such reassuring words. 'The lesson we should learn from diseases such as BSE and indeed Aids is that there are other agents out there which can cross the species barrier and which are very real problems,' says Malcolm Eames. 'It is not good enough to screen for diseases that we are aware of. Other viruses exist in host species that we are not aware of and cannot test for until they have crossed the species barrier. Breeding pigs in a germ-free environment cannot absolutely rule out a new disease emerging and crossing that barrier.'

Serious doubts have also been raised about the reliability and safety of the technology of genetic engineering. White and

Wallwork might only be engineering lowly pigs, but the anti-vivisection movement raises the spectre of Frankenstein to condemn those who experiment with the genetic structure of animals. 'The technology has been shown to cause considerable suffering and distress to a large number of animals,' says Eames. 'There is considerable evidence that this unreliable technique often has horrendous physical, psychological and behavioural side effects on the animals used. One well-known example was the attempt to genetically engineer a super-pig in a US government research station. The human growth hormone was genetically incorporated into the pig to produce a fast-growing animal. The pigs suffered from defective vision, stomach ulcers, muscular weakness, arthritis, impotence and lethargy. Some had deformed skulls.'

John Wallwork is combative in the face of such criticisms. The genetic engineers who produced the deformed animals should have known better, he says, and could easily have predicted the results before they began. He thinks such anxieties are rooted in ignorance. 'I think the public are concerned about Frankenstein-ian doctors making crazy animals that are going to think like man,' he explains. 'I think that's reasonable if you don't understand genetics and medicine, and we've been trying over the years to explain and to inform the public what we are up to. We are not tinkering and we are very interested in animal welfare. We are not interested in producing pigs that are deformed or indeed suffering. That's of no value to us at all, to have sick pigs. As far as we are aware from all our tests, they are indistinguishable on a normal biological level from ordinary pigs. They breed normally, they look normal, they eat normally, they live normally and they are normal pigs. Now if they were in some way made sickly then obviously our research wouldn't be able to continue because it wouldn't be sensible and we wouldn't want to do it. There's a hard core of people who will object to anything. There's a hard core that objected to television, to blood transfusions, to the motor car. But what we are trying to do is deal with the mass of the population who think it is sensible to help people who are sick. That's the bottom line.'

White adds scientific weight to this defence. He says that the insertion of the human 'flag' into his genetically engineered pigs has altered their basic structure by one millionth of 1 per cent and cannot possibly have any deleterious effects on the animals. 'It's trivial,' he says. 'You can get that by a series of mutations on any farm on any day of the week. So what we are doing is a very precise piece of genetic engineering. We go to an awful lot of trouble and expense to know what we are doing. I fully understand the anxieties of people who are concerned about tinkering with nature. But, quite frankly, people would rather be alive than dead. And if you go and talk with people who are waiting for a heart transplant, they know perfectly well that their chances of getting a heart are probably no more than fifty-fifty. You ask them whether they think it's a good idea or a bad idea to do this work. They are the people who count.'

White and Wallwork have not been put off, either by the angry words or by the violence. They believe the protests will be short-lived once their pigs begin to save lives. But will it be a heart from one of their pigs or someone else's that first begins to beat inside a human chest? The two Englishmen are no longer the only people to dream of ending the donor shortage with animal organs. They are now in a race with an American biotechnology company called Alexion Pharmaceuticals in New Haven, Connecticut, that has its own herd of genetically engineered pigs[31] and is vying for the pot of gold that will reward the group that first makes animal organs work in humans. The pace is picking up.

In April 1995, a genetically engineered pig belonging to Alexion Pharmaceuticals was anaesthetized and wheeled into an experimental operating theatre in New York. A team of surgeons removed its liver and one of its lungs and preserved them with ice while two baboons were prepared for surgery on adjoining operating tables. The organs were then transplanted into the monkeys. One of the pig's kidneys was also removed and later transplanted into a third baboon. This was one of several experimental operations that the two firms have been under-taking to test the viability of their genetically engineered organs. They have taken place at secret locations with tight security and little publicity, to avoid the kind of reprisals that David White suffered at his home. A baboon's body would react, the experimenters believe, in much the same way as a person's in the presence of a transplanted pig's organ. If the genetically engineered organs are not hyperacutely rejected when transplanted into baboons, they should not be rejected when they are put into humans. That, at least, is the theory, and the experimenters say that the first results from their second-generation pigs have been encouraging. They have been comparing the time it takes a baboon to reject a genetically engineered pig's organ with the time it takes it to reject a normal pig's organ. Hyperacute rejection would usually destroy a pig's organ within about two hours. Alexion says that their engineered organs have been surviving in baboons for as long as two days without immuno-suppression. But Imutran claims the most dramatic improvements. They have been transplanting engineered pigs' hearts into the abdomens of monkeys: 'One of our transgenic pig hearts . . . will survive for about as long as if it were a monkey heart – about five and a half days,' explains David White. 'We've gone on from there, of course, and immuno-suppressed the monkeys and now we can get pigs' hearts to work in primates for months. We don't know how long yet as those experiments are still on-going.'

Ultimately, the winners of this high-technology race might not be the team that first puts a pig's heart into a person but, rather, the team that wins the legal battle to exploit the fruits of their labours. So far, the competition betweeen Imutran and Alexion has been conducted in a gentlemanly and good-humoured fashion, but with big institutional money now backing both companies and with such large sums at stake, the race could turn nasty. In 1989, David White filed a patent on his genetic-engineering technique, that's already been granted in several countries. He believes America and Europe will do likewise in 1996. If it is granted in the USA it could block Alexion's hopes of reaping a whirlwind profit from their engineered pigs. Alexion Pharmaceuticals entered the race nine years after Imutran, but has also applied for a world-wide patent for its complement inhibitor. As the two companies edge closer to the clinic, all the signs are that a bitter courtroom battle lies ahead.

'The details of who claims what in these patents will be critical,' says Alexion's President, Leonard Bell. 'So far, of the two firms, only Alexion has a patent granted in the US. We expect that the potential conflicts will clarify themselves as the success of the various techniques becomes more clear.'

White is confident that Imutran is well ahead of the pack, if only because he was the first to begin breeding genetically engineered pigs and it takes a fixed time to raise such animals to maturity. And if the experimental transplants continue to bear out the theories, the first clinical trials are not far away. 'We have to be absolutely sure we've got the science right before we start transplanting human beings,' he says, '. . . [but] at the end of the day we've got to have the courage to say: "Yes, we have done everything we can do; we believe the science is right and we've got to start undertaking clinical trials." It's not there yet, but it's coming closer. The first clinical trials may take place in 1997 but it's going to take perhaps five years before pigs are available generally for transplantation. We are talking very much about the future here.'

The question is, of course, what kind of future is on offer? Is it a future in which high-technology medicine comes to the rescue of young babies born with congenitally defective organs? Perhaps. But such victims of fate and circumstance will only ever be a small proportion of the burgeoning demand for transplanted organs. If the immunological problems can be overcome, we are much more likely to see animal organs used increasingly to repair the damage that our own short-sighted lifestyles have wrought on our bodies. Poor diet, lack of exercise, smoking, drinking, pollution and over-stressed Western lives are responsible for a high proportion of the diseases for which transplant surgery holds out the promise of a cure. But do we want to make doctors into pit-stop human-body mechanics – specialists who remove the organs we destroy with our frantic, self-centred lives, replacing them with new ones so that we can continue in our self-destructive ways? Or should the real role of the medical practitioner be to advise the rest of us how to be healthy and happy and how to avoid the need for animal organ transplants later on in life? Wouldn't preventive medicine be a better use of scarce resources than ploughing money into pig's organs?

'Animals are not the answer to disease and the problems of the human condition,' insists Dr Moneim Fadali, a cardiac surgeon from Los Angeles in California who strongly opposed Leonard Bailey's decision to transplant a baboon heart into Baby Fae in 1984. 'According to our national cancer institute, 80 per cent of cancers are preventable. The same is almost true with heart disease. So we are abdicating our responsibility for our own destiny by using other species in order to correct the misuse of our lives and nature. . . . It's about time we rose above our egocentricity. That is bad. The end result is not good for humanity. It is disastrous for humanity.'

8

Brave New Bodies

At a black-tie ceremony in Cleveland, Ohio, in April 1988, Robert J. White, a distinguished American neurosurgeon, received two contrasting awards. The first was given in recognition of his lifelong contribution to medicine: he was nominated National Health Professional of the Year by the Visiting Nurses Association. The second had a different ring to it: he was named Vivisector of the Year by Sherry Hamilton, an animal rights activist who stormed onto the podium during the ceremony to condemn Robert White as an 'embarrassment to the human species'. As security guards hustled her off the stage, she added a few more words to the citation. 'We speak for those who cannot – so they are not forgotten,' she shouted. 'The millions of animals killed in agony. For inhumanity surpassing all others in your field.'[1]

Robert White had earned this dubious accolade for conducting experiments that, he hoped, would one day make him the first surgeon to transplant an entire human body onto a severed human head. If this sounds like the sales pitch for a 1950s horror movie, don't be fooled. Dr White is serious about his desire to turn science fiction into science fact. That is, after all, the story of transplant surgery over the past fifty years. The boundaries of the possible have repeatedly been pushed ever further into the unknown. In 1950 surgeons could not transplant a kidney. Today, an Englishman owes his life to the six new organs he received in 1994. Why *not* transplant a human body onto a human head? This is, of course, as much an ethical question as a practical one: it might be technically possible, but is it desirable? After all, the lesson of the atomic era is only too clear: we might have the ability to explode hugely destructive weapons, but the world community has decided that this isn't a sensible thing to do. How far should we take the developing technology of transplant surgery? Robert White has a clear vision of the future. He believes whole-body transplants will one day be as acceptable a cure for certain diseases as heart, liver and kidney transplants are today. He has spent several years testing the idea on animals in the laboratories at Case Western Reserve University.

'When we first undertook the experiments, I intrinsically felt that this accomplishment would, in certain quarters, be looked upon as a Frankensteinian undertaking,' says White. 'No matter how hard I argued that it had great importance and potential in terms of human disease, there would always be a group which would have totally opposed the development and undertaking of those experiments.'

He was right. The first reaction to the idea of transplanting an entire body onto a head is disbelieving mirth. The notion is dismissed as nonsense – a bad joke. When the technique is shown to be a practical possibility, scepticism and laughter turn to horror. 'He must be mad' is the common response. But Robert White is no lunatic. He is a humorous, intelligent man, a Catholic who has a strong belief in the morality of his work. The walls of his office on the ninth floor of the Hamann Building in the university's Metrohealth Centre are covered with photographic mementoes of his meetings with Pope John Paul II for whom he acts as an adviser on ethical matters. He has written over 600 medical and scientific publications dealing with clinical neurology, medical ethics and brain research. He's been the President of Cleveland's Academy of Medicine and has served as editor or on the editorial board of four respected academic journals. He has also received several honorary doctorate degrees and was named Ohio Neurosurgeon of the year in 1983. With such a background it is perhaps all the more surprising to find Robert White working in a field that provokes such angry indignation.

'The details of his experiments are so horrifying that they seem to reach the limits of scientific depravity,' was the response of Catherine Roberts, the scientist, author and anti-vivisectionist, when she first heard about his work.[2]

White's unusual experiments grew out of neurological research he conducted on monkeys early in the 1960s. He wanted to find out if low temperature was an effective means of treating brains that had been injured or had suffered strokes. He also hoped to discover whether this technique could help protect the brain when its blood supply was interrupted during an operation. To do so he needed to reproduce the phenomenon experimentally. There was, he decided, only one way to do this.

'The first steps taken were to remove the brain from the cranium [the skull] of a monkey,'[3] explains White, 'and maintain it alive on a mechanical circuit that had an artificial heart, an artificial lung and, of course, tubing that would be the equivalent of blood vessels. . . . By being able to study these various phenomena under the total control of the investigator, I think we can really stretch and expand our understanding of the brain.'

Visitors to White's laboratory in the 1960s would have been confronted with a living brain held in a metal support, its vital functions sustained by tubes and pumps and its surface covered with wires and electrodes. The guests could have been forgiven for thinking they had stepped into a movie set, but Robert White would not take kindly to such a parallel: like many academics, the scientific jargon that he uses in reports of his experiments tends to obscure the emotional impact of his work, in much the same way that during the Cold War the military talked of 'megadeaths', when they meant mass killing of millions, and 'collateral damage', when they meant the slaughter of innocent civilians. In this vein, Robert White talks fondly of his 'brain models' and his 'preparations' when he means the removal of the brain from the skull of a Rhesus monkey and keeping it alive artificially. Not even the head of the animal escapes this linguistic mutilation. In White's language, it is transformed into a 'cephalon'.

On 17 January 1962 he achieved his objective of isolating a monkey's brain, supplying it with oxygen-rich blood to preserve its functions. He isolated several brains in this way. Throughout these experiments, he assumed the brains were in a deep sleep, but the electric impulses they generated sometimes suggested wakefulness. A new question entered his mind: the brains might be alive on a neurological level, but are they conscious? Are they still aware of their own existence? As he had severed all the brains' connections with the outside world, removing their eyes, ears, nose, tongue and all the sensations they would normally have received from the body, this proved difficult to answer. It came to dominate his thinking, and the attempt to answer it motivated his desire to transplant whole bodies onto severed heads. The first step along that path was a second series of experiments with isolated monkey brains. This time, when White removed the brain, he preserved the nerve leading to one of the eyes or to the eardrum and middle-ear structures. By placing electrodes on the surface of the isolated brain to record its activity, and electrically stimulating the optic or auditory nerves, he demonstrated that it was still responsive to sound or light. It was tantalizing, but it still didn't answer the central question.

'People said: "Well, that's wonderful, and the brain-waves look very good and the chemistry is very exciting. It looks normal – but how do we know that the brain is thinking? Does it have consciousness? Does it have memory? And so forth." In a sense it would be impossible to answer that question with just a transplant of the brain itself. And so I thought: "Well, if we leave the brain inside the skull and then transplant a body to it, wouldn't it be possible to expect that brain . . . to regain consciousness, to be able to hear, taste, smell, feel?'

To sever a monkey's head from its body and then reconnect it to the headless torso of another monkey, Robert White had to devise new surgical techniques and a new form of anaesthesia. He also had to construct a sophisticated suspension frame to hold the body and head of his 'preparations'. In the 1970s and 1980s he led a team of surgeons that performed up to thirty successful total body transplants. He calls them head transplants although it is clear that the body is being given to the head and not the other way round. The first was in March 1970. 'I must confess that we failed a number of times,' says White. 'But when one of these head transplants awakened, after all those weeks of failure, there was dancing, there was singing. Why, I think the hospital almost fell down that particular evening that we had our first successful head transplant. This animal was not only awake, it would track you with its eyes as you walked round the laboratory and could hear noises and voices and was very irritable. As a matter of fact, to check somebody put their finger inside the mouth and it was nearly bitten off.'[4]

White had proved that consciousness could be transplanted. But the monkey wasn't singing and dancing along with its human captors. It had woken up to discover its head attached to a body it did not recognize and over which it had no control. The poor beast was paralysed from the neck down because it was (and still is) impossible to join its spinal cord – the neural highway that links head and body – to the cord in the body of the donor. It couldn't even breathe unaided.[5] So, while the donor's heart pumped blood through the arteries and veins in the recipient's head, the life of this surgical hybrid ultimately rested on a ventilator forcing air into lungs that no longer worked on their own. From the monkey's perspective, it was perhaps fortunate that White didn't have the funds to take care of the animals for long. Once rejection took its toll and the monkeys' faces started to swell and bleed, they were killed. None lived longer than a week after its operation. He claims that the animals were not in pain during their short experimental lives as his medical team used liberal doses of local anaesthetic to prevent any physical discomfort. But one can only wonder at the psychological effects of the operation on the recipient.

'The sensations experienced by these minds are unimaginably horrifying,' writes Hans Ruesch, a medical historian and leader of an anti-vivisectionist movement called Civitas. 'It is not simply a situation of confusion, distress or shock such as suffered by an appallingly mutilated but still living animal: it is a situation of artificially imposed amplification of pain, or other terrifying sensations, from which the natural relief mechanism has been disconnected. Under conditions of extreme pain or mortal fear an intact animal will faint or become comatose through loss of blood supply to the brain. But this release from pain and fear is not available to the heads fed by machines or donors. The pump goes on whatever the brain's sensations and whatever the level of pain.'[6]

Inevitably, the animal rights movement did their best to make

Robert White's life a misery for conducting research that would turn the stomachs of all but the most hardened observers. 'I don't think I was prepared for the overwhelming uproar that occurred when those experiments first became known to the public,' White recalls. 'I had a lot of criticism: oh, disturbing death threats, my children were threatened and called the most abusive language, my daughters particularly. There was at least one break-in at the university where attempts were made to destroy equipment and files. The bottom line is that I required a great deal of protection and was given it by the FBI, the Secret Service, the local and suburban police. So for a period of time I was under a lot of attack from the animal rights groups, particularly in this country.'

Robert White had stirred up a hornets' nest of protest to prove that he could transplant consciousness. It seemed like a lot of trouble for a rather dubious intellectual gain. Wasn't this just experimentation for the sheer sake of it? Wasn't it science devoid of an ethical context, the same amoral motive that has made so many intelligent people devote their lives to the perfection of weapons of mass destruction? At first sight, those who condemn Robert White as either mad or bad appear to have right firmly on their side. His work is certainly outside the mainstream of transplant surgery. But the moral issues become cloudier if you duck the instant condemnation and delve beneath the surface. White is not plagued by his conscience. He believes that if it is right to save someone's life with a transplanted organ, it is just as right to do the same with a transplanted body. He even has the blessing of the Catholic Church. 'While I may have been having trouble with the animal rights groups in the world, certainly my own religious leaders have been very supportive of my work,' he says. 'They know there have been spin-offs from this transplantation work that have to do with the care of the injured brain.'

The problem, Robert White believes, is of perception. Transplanted organs are acceptable because hearts, livers and kidneys are placed inside the body and are therefore hidden from view. The idea of a transplanted body produces such strong negative emotions because it is there for all to see. 'What if we could transplant an arm or a leg successfully?' says White. 'I think that the public might be very concerned and think: "Well, that's a dead arm and now it's alive because it's on somebody!" And I think exactly the same problem is present when you're talking about a body or a head transplant. You can see this thing and people can almost visualize: "Where's that poor person's body gone?" or "Where has the head gone that was on the body before?" So I think a lot of it is imagery. We've got to get away from the idea that because we're transplanting the entire body there's something very special about that over transplanting a set of lungs and a heart.'

White sees the body as little more than a 'power-pack' dedicated to the survival of the head, the seat of consciousness. Viewed in that light, the difference between an organ transplant and a whole body transplant is purely quantitative. Even if one was to accept such reasoning – and it ignores the fact that we express our personalities through the subtleties of body language as much as we do with facial expressions and the spoken word – there is a still more fundamental objection to the idea of whole body transplants. Until surgeons learn how to reconnect the millions of nerves of the spinal cord, the head would be unable to move a muscle of its new body. It couldn't breathe for itself. It couldn't speak. It couldn't move its new arms and legs. Who in their right mind would want a body that requires twenty-four-hour-a-day medical attention to survive? Robert White even has an answer to this: his work at the Metro Health Centre brings him into regular contact with quadriplegics – people who have lost the use of their limbs as a result of traumatic accidents that damage or sever their spinal cords. 'They die much sooner than somebody who doesn't have this form of injury,' says White, 'and they die because of multi-organ failure. In other words they are probably twenty or thirty or more years short of the average of a normal man or woman. So the issue is on the board immediately. What are we supposed to do? They're not a candidate for a multi-organ transplant because their whole body is failing . . . and their doctor comes to us and says: "Could you give him a new body?" And the answer is, "Sure." Do I have any reservations on a moral or ethical basis for doing this or wishing that it could be done? The answer is no, because I believe first and foremost we are attempting to extend life through the advantages of the human brain.'

Is this just an idle dream? Would a paralysed person take up White's offer? Forty-three-year-old Craig Vetovitz is in a good position to put the hypothesis to the test. He broke his neck in a swimming accident in 1971 and has suffered from quadriplegia ever since. 'Back in June 1971 on Father's Day, two friends and I were swimming in the backyard pool,' Craig recalls from his home in Medina, Ohio. 'Like most guys we were just clowning around and towards the end of the afternoon we were getting pretty tired. When I did my dive I hit the water the wrong way because I could not execute the right posture. My head hit the water first. It shoved my chin directly into my chest. I felt something in my neck snap and that's the last I remember. Oh, for four weeks I was out of it.'

When Craig came to he was unable to move anything beneath the level of his chin. The transition from a fit athlete to a bedridden, helpless patient was unimaginably traumatic. 'Some days you'd be burning up from inside out,' he says. 'Five minutes later you'd be freezing to death. You cannot sit up. You have holes drilled in your skull. You have traction put in. You are humiliated. You feel you've lost all self-respect, because at that first point, the rude awakening is being dependent upon someone to help you run and lead your life. You cannot describe that feeling. It's totally the worst nightmare that anybody could ever imagine.'

Fortunately Craig hadn't severed his spinal cord but it had been seriously damaged. As the years passed he regained a little movement and sensation in his limbs. This was as much of a curse as it was a blessing: he is now in permanent pain. He still cannot walk, stand unaided or use his hands. He requires constant assistance for the most basic personal activities. But Craig runs a polymer engineering business from his wheelchair and wants to live. His work gives him a strong sense of fulfilment, he has plans and goals for the future, and if his body begins to fail he would jump at the chance of a total body transplant. 'Right now I am forty-three years of age. I have a lot going for me in my life. Most physically challenged people want their life to end. I'm not ready for that yet. I can feel my body ageing. I can feel my endurance lessening. I feel the pain more often and, yes, if I could have a transplant of this sort that would enable me to live longer . . . I'm all for it. Not only for my own dream but for my own personal goals – to help the people out who have helped me and backed me.'

The pleas of quadriplegics like Craig Vetovitz are hard to ignore. They have as much right to life as the person dying of liver or heart disease. If a whole-body transplant could prolong their lives, are they to be denied it because the rest of us find the idea distasteful? The long-term problems of rejection in a whole-body transplant are still unknown: the experiments to determine this have still to be undertaken. But Craig thinks White's work should continue, and he has little time for those who raise moral objections. 'Before they have any right to say it's wrong or it's cruel, they've got to do two things,' he says. 'One: they should spend many months in a specialized children's hospital seeing children who are born with a disability or who have acquired one through an accident, and let them see the suffering that child is going through. Let them experience it, hands on. Let them experience the grief the parents are going through. Let them really see and feel it. And the second thing they should do is be injected with drugs to put them in a quadriplegic state so they cannot move from their shoulders down for six months. Let them use a wheelchair. Let them endure the elements we have to. When they do that, then I feel they have the right to make an honest opinion. Until then they should shut up.'

Ultimately, Craig sees Robert White's whole-body transplant as a beacon of hope, which would give him a chance to stay alive long enough for neurologists to discover a way of repairing his spinal cord and restoring the mobility he so desperately craves. That day might not be far away, although it will probably not come as soon as Craig hopes.

'My predication,' says Robert White, 'would be that certainly within the next fifty years – which isn't much longer than we've already gone through with organ transplantation – we will be able to grow the spinal cord back together again in the injured patient. Now, if we can do that, then if you do a body transplant it should be eminently possible to grow the cord from the brain to the new body's spinal cord. Under those circumstances, this operation would offer the patient's brain the possibility of regaining control and use of the body.'

Robert White's dream of being the first surgeon to transplant an entire body onto a human head will not come true in America. He feels that ethical qualms would prevent him from doing such an operation in his own country. He has thought of exporting his vision to the Ukraine where, he believes, he will have less trouble with what he regards as armchair moralists. 'I have considered doing it in Kiev,' he says. 'They have an outstanding neurosurgical centre. They have very fine surgeons – but they are poor. So I thought that I would be able to outfit their operating and intensive care rooms and . . . [then] could fly someone in . . . and do the operation there. I think the moral and ethical issues would be less of a concern in the Ukraine than they would be here.'

Whatever the benefits to quadriplegics, the future that White conjures up is strange: human beings who cheat death by changing their bodies when the old one packs up; a world populated by whole-body transplantees on their second, third or fourth bodies; ageing heads walking on young and vital limbs. Such a nightmare scenario might be a distant fantasy, but it is the logical conclusion of Robert White's work. He speaks earnestly about the medical benefits of the technique: 'We're not talking about extending people's lives who are eighty and ninety and so forth,' he says. 'We're talking about young people whose total body has failed.' But in the next breath he's talking passionately about immortality. 'Could the brain live for ever?' he wonders. 'In a sense, its ageing may indeed reflect the fact that the other organs are deteriorating. Since we now have ways of replacing them – and perhaps even the whole body – does it mean that if the brain were to receive all of the proper nutrients . . . that immortality would be built into the nerve cells? I think that's a possibility. A lot of people would disagree with it but . . . I really think there should be ways of protecting the brain from that sort of cellular disintegration.'

Surgeons like Robert White who desire to push the boundaries of spare-part surgery ever outwards are motivated by two separate agendas. One, above-board, obvious and honourable is the desire to save the lives of desperately ill patients. The other, buried deep in the collective twentieth-century mind, is an unsettling sense of our own mortality, the fear of death. It is hard to escape the conclusion that we have become so divorced from the natural process of life and death, so wrapped up in our Western materialist dream, that we now secretly desire physical immortality and would, if we could, use whole-body transplantation to delay indefinitely the day of reckoning. The technology of spare-part surgery might be a blessing for thousands of desperately ill patients, but it is also a reflection of the spiritual vacuum at the heart of our culture. Already, the line between a reasonable attempt to save life and a desperate one to cheat death is very fine.

Laura Davies was born at St Mary's Hospital in Manchester in April 1988 with a rare, life-threatening disorder of her bowel called gastroschisis. Much of her small and large intestines were missing and the section that was present had developed outside her body, thanks to a hole in her abdominal wall near her navel. Without surgery she would have lived at most for a few days. But if surgeons had removed her defective bowel, she would have been unable to digest food and could only have been kept alive by being fed through an intravenous tube. Laura's parents, Les and Frances, could have decided to let their baby die, but after talking to their doctors they embarked on a five-year struggle to keep her alive. By 1993 the little girl with the smiling face and golden curls was known all over Britain and America. The ups and downs of Laura's condition, her endless hospital visits, the life-saving operations, including two major transplants, were all subjected to obsessive scrutiny. Today, the decision to prolong her life has come to haunt her father.

'Looking back, if I knew then what I know now I wouldn't even have had the first bowel operation,' says a bitter Les Davies from his home in Manchester. 'It's like a production line. They're pushing them all the time to see how much life they can get out of them – what more they can do to keep them alive . . . We decided no. Enough is enough.'

Laura Davies's life was perpetually balanced on a knife-edge. The complications of the treatments she needed to stay alive were always threatening to tip her into the abyss. As time went on, her body became weaker and the unwanted side effects increasingly difficult to control. When she was three and a half she developed a severe chest infection and spent eight weeks in intensive care on a ventilator. A few months later, in 1992, her face turned yellow when her liver failed. Laura's doctors said her only hope was an experimental double-organ transplant, which Sir Roy Calne, the British transplant pioneer, offered to do. The family said no. They had heard that the Americans had more experience with such operations and were also using a promising new drug called FK506. They launched an appeal for money to send their daughter to the Children's Hospital in Pittsburgh and had soon raised £350,000, thanks to the generosity of the British public and King Fahd of Saudi Arabia, who supplied £150,000.

In May 1992, Laura and her parents flew to Pittsburgh where, less than two weeks later, she was given a new liver and small bowel, followed by a further operation to stem blood-flow. Les and Frances waited anxiously by their daughter's bedside as she slowly recovered.

In November, they all flew back to Manchester, where Laura was the toast of the town. Three months later, she was back in Pittsburgh having a swollen spleen removed, and as spring turned into summer Laura's doctors began to lose their hold on her precarious health. She developed cancer-like growths in her intestines, caused by a virus that the FK506 and other anti-rejection drugs had allowed to grow unchecked. The dosage was reduced but then the transplanted intestines failed as Laura's body began to reject the new organs. The medical team was chasing its tail. Their patient stopped eating and in September 1993 she was back on the transplant waiting list, her internal organs so badly affected by the drug treatment that her life could be saved only by transplanting six new organs into her: a liver, stomach, pancreas, small intestine, bowel and kidney. It was a step too far for many opinionated writers in the British press. Sympathy for Laura turned into a savage attack on her doctors, who were accused of prolonging the agony of a young child to advance medical knowledge.

'There is something very distasteful,' complained Margaret Maxwell in the *Independent*, 'about subjecting tiny children to operations that are at the very frontier of medical competence and require such invasive and massive surgery . . . She seems to have been sucked into a terrible round of operations and treatments in which recovery is illusory.'[7]

Melanie Phillips, the *Observer*'s correspondent, was just as harsh: 'Underpinning the whole march of experimentation and medical advance is a collective self-delusion,' she wrote. 'It is that advances in medical technology remove suffering and can even cheat death itself. . . . Indeed, one wonders whether what is driving her doctors on is not so much the desire to end physical suffering but the excitement of scientists on the frontiers of research. . . . Extraordinary efforts to cheat nature are not only pointless but rob human life of its dignity.'[8]

It was, of course, much easier to carp on the sidelines than to be in the driving seat in Pittsburgh taking the difficult decisions. Andreas Tzakis, Laura's surgeon, believed he could save her with six new organs. He had already given twelve other patients multi-transplants and had reason for his optimism: eight were still alive. Tzakis had not put in as many as six before, but he had the full backing of Laura's parents.

'What do people expect us to do? Just pull out the tubes, stop the drugs and leave her to die?' an angry Les Davies told the press. 'If they could see her they would know that you can't give up on her. This child is living . . . and the people here love and care for her and wouldn't put her through anything if they did not feel it would give her a chance.'[9]

For now, mother and father were united in the belief that they were doing the right thing. 'There is a chance she will live,' said Frances Davies. 'If we don't take that chance, Laura will die. How can we take that chance away from her? It would be murder. If she was really critically ill, it might be different, but she's mentally alert and active. She doesn't feel pain at the moment and doesn't seem to remember her previous operation. She's not giving up, why should we?'[10]

On 16 September the Pittsburgh medical team found a donor and, with the eyes of the world watching her, the little girl from Manchester underwent her second major transplant operation in fifteen months. She was too young to appreciate it, but when she woke up from the anaesthetic, Laura Davies had attained a unique status in the medical world: the only person alive whose existence now depended on six transplanted organs. It was a distinction which few would envy and one that she did not hold for long. The narrow ledge that Laura's doctors had been treading between infection and rejection had become a knife-edge as the combined effects of major surgery and powerful drugs began to overwhelm her frail body. In October her left lung collapsed, a delayed effect of the anaesthetic she needed during the sixteen-hour operation. By the middle of November, the anti-rejection drug FK506 had again so weakened her immune system that her body was no longer able to recognize abnormal cells. Small cancer-like growths invaded her intestines as they had after her first transplant. Laura was in the intensive care ward breathing with the assistance of a ventilator when she suffered a stroke. Her distraught parents decided that enough was enough. But some of the medical team thought they should be given one more chance to save Laura's life, another week of life-support in the hope of finding a way of reversing her terminal decline. It was a step too far for Laura's father.

'At the end . . . they started bringing in a kidney dialysis machine to keep her going,' he explains. 'They would have liked to have kept her alive to see what else they could have got from her. That part of it is bang out of order . . . There is no way I would let them keep her alive a week longer when it was clear she had no chance. I feel angry about that. When they know it's gone too far and there is no hope left, they are professionals and they should call a halt. There is no respect for life – to let children go to the lengths they did and using the parents, because parents don't have enough information and are blinded by hope.'

Laura's mother insisted that the doctors allow her to die. 'I realized there was nothing we could do to save her,' she explained at the time. 'I refused to let them hook her back to the [dialysis] machine. They were saying they could still turn her around. It was my choice. We said to the doctors: "Let's do it now." I didn't want her to suffer any more. I could never have lived with myself if I thought her pain was being prolonged.'[11]

Laura's ventilator was switched off on 11 November 1993. The long struggle to save her life, which had seemed so worthwhile at the time, had ended in bitterness and despair. Les and Frances Davies's marriage broke down. Les lives alone now – plagued by his memories of Laura and what he now sees as the unnecessary suffering caused by the extraordinary efforts to save her life. 'Maybe we would have been better off fifty years ago,' he says, 'when they would have said: "There's nothing we can do for Laura now but let her die." She would not have had to go through all that – two different operations, infections, intensive-care units. That's not quality of life.'

Laura's surgeon, Andreas Tzakis, has been chastened by the experience. He has learnt that the sophisticated technology of transplant surgery can sometimes prevent doctors from appreciating the limits to medical intervention. It takes courage to say no, to advise relatives that it may be better to let a patient die peacefully than to prolong their suffering in the vain hope of snatching victory from the jaws of death. But knowing when to refuse treatment and when to continue the fight is a finely balanced decision.

'We failed,' says Tzakis, 'and, in retrospect, perhaps we should not have attempted the second transplant. We knew that the chances were poor, but we were fighting for her life. So yes, if you want to say it, the critics were right. But at other times we have been right and they have been wrong. It is not an all-or-nothing phenomenon. Our work causes controversy because it is experimental and difficult decisions have to be made . . . Would I do the same thing again? Having failed, it would be arrogant of me to say, yes, I would do it again. Of course not. If we had known it was going to fail, we would not have done it.'

Laura Davies was five and a half when she died. It is tempting to see the dogged determination to save her life as an understandable overreaction by her doctors and parents and not as an example of a modern malaise. Surely such a situation would never arise with an older person, someone able to express their own opinion about their treatment? Wouldn't doctors and relatives defer to the patient's wishes – even if that meant allowing them to die? Just a few months after Laura's death, Andreas Tzakis (who was now working at the Jackson Memorial Hospital in Miami) and the transplant team at Pittsburgh Children's Hospital were embroiled in another similar controversy. Benito Agrelo, a teenager, suffered such severe side effects from his anti-rejection medication that he decided to stop taking the drugs and let nature take its course. If he died, he reasoned, at least he would have enjoyed a few months of good quality life. The hospital's response made it clear that the Laura Davies episode was far from an exception. They had Benito forcibly seized from his home in Coral Springs, near Miami, strapped to a stretcher and driven to hospital in an attempt to make him take the drugs. Even the police who helped manhandle the patient into an ambulance were disturbed by the incident. 'When I look back on the entire thing,' says Detective Charles Amos of Coral Springs police station in Florida, 'I still have a very sick feeling in my stomach. I think, as a police officer, I did not help . . . Benny at all. It makes me feel very sick.'

Benito Agrelo was born in 1979 with a hereditary disease called alpha-antitrypsin deficiency, the most common genetic cause of liver disease in children.[12] By the time he was nine his health had so deteriorated that his skin had turned yellow, discoloured by the toxins that his liver could no longer remove from his body. A transplant was Benito's only hope, and in May 1988 he was given a new liver by Andreas Tzakis at Pittsburgh Children's Hospital. He lived a normal life for the next four years, his new liver protected from the destructive effects of his immune system by daily doses of Cyclosporin. As ever, the medical balancing act was imperfect: powerful drugs slowed the rejection process but, as the years passed, the efficient functioning of Benito's new liver was slowly undermined. When he was thirteen he was as sick as he had been at nine. He needed a second transplant, given to him by Jorge Reyes, another surgeon at the Pittsburgh Hospital. Benito had recovered rapidly from the first, but this time, in December 1992, his weakened body took a terrible beating. 'While he was in intensive care,' remembers Claudine Com, a close friend of Benito's, 'he started to bleed internally so they rushed him back into the emergency room and did another major operation and then brought him back into intensive care. But he started bleeding again and went in for more surgery. They'd stapled him under his arms instead of stitching him, and whenever he moved just a little bit he would tear a staple and start to bleed again. Then when he was doing a little better and was back up in his room, he would have these seizures. He had three of them and each time he had one he'd wake up back down in intensive care again not knowing why he was there or what had happened. He endured an awful lot of pain.'

Because Cyclosporin had failed to prevent his body from rejecting the first transplant, Benito was placed on FK506. Clinical tests had shown it to be even more effective than Cyclosporin at combating rejection in transplanted livers,[13] and his doctors hoped it would prove just as potent inside his ailing body. Benito recovered from his operation and left Pittsburgh hospital with healthy pink skin and a liver that, thanks to FK506 and various other anti-rejection medications, was doing the job it was meant to do. There was a heavy cost, however. Benito's life had been saved – but now it was made unbearable by the side effects of the drugs: blinding headaches forced him to lie down with the lights turned off; his back and legs ached and he was short of breath, which prevented him from being with his friends; he was always tired and suffered frequent bouts of vomiting. The endless suffering brought him to a cross-roads in his life: he took a decision that plunged his family and the transplant teams at the hospitals in Pittsburgh and Miami into the deepest controversy. The first people he told were Claudine Com and his brother, Frank, after a visit to Disneyworld. They'd rented a wheelchair to prevent Benito from becoming too tired and had planned the trip with military precision – carrying with them syringes, cups and various drugs and ensured that he stopped periodically to take his medicines at the proper time. Benito broke the news to them as they drove home.

'We had been driving for a while and just talking about life in general,' says Com. 'Benny had just commented, matter-of-factly, that he was sick and tired of all the medication and his legs being swollen all the time and the headaches and everything else. He wanted to live a normal life without working to a schedule, just doing things when he felt like doing them. He no longer wanted to take the medication or go to the hospitals to have all the tests done any more. He just wanted to enjoy life as it came. It was more a statement of fact. It wasn't like he was looking for my opinion on it. It was like he had thought about it for a real long time and he was finally saying out loud words that he'd thought about for a while.'

This was hardly surprising. Benito Agrelo had lived for years with severe pain and suffering and was now unable to live the life of a normal teenager. He couldn't go dancing. He couldn't date girls and had to spend long hours at home nursing his sick body. In these circumstances he could be forgiven for succumbing to gloom in considering a course of action that would end in his death. Kind words and loving attention might have dissuaded most young children from taking such a drastic decision. But the depths of Benito's suffering had matured him beyond his years. Those who saw him remarked on his clarity of vision, his self-possession and his grace. He had not come to this conclusion lightly. He knew that a decision to stop taking the drugs would be signing his own death warrant. But he had decided that the quality of his life was too poor to wish to continue it. Rather a few months of good health followed by a slide into oblivion than decades of continual suffering. That was Benito's view and no one could shift him from it, not even his mother.

'She talked to Benny for a long time when he made the decision not to take the medication,' says Claudine. 'She wasn't sure which was the right way to go. It was a long process [but] she knew her son, and she supported him 100 per cent. It was his way of saying:

"I want to try to do this by God's wishes. Let God guide my life and if I'm meant to live a long life, then I will – and if not, then I won't." And his mum understood that and stood behind him.'

Benito stopped taking his anti-rejection medicines in October 1993, ten months after his second transplant. The side effects disappeared and for the first time in years Benito found himself free of pain. For a few months he led the kind of life that most fifteen-year-olds take for granted.

'It was phenomenal when he stopped taking the medication,' Claudine explains. 'He was doing everything he wanted to do. He drove me crazy – every day . . . We went all over the place. He had energy and he was always happy and everything was OK, you know, nothing hurt any more. He didn't have the leg aches and the headaches and was able to take the long walks that he always liked to take. And he was eating! I couldn't believe the amount of food he could consume.'

Benito described the nine months after he stopped taking his drugs in October 1993 as 'the best months of my life'.[14] But by June 1994 his skin had started to take on a characteristic yellow hue, the first outward sign that, without the protection of immuno-suppressant drugs, his body was destroying his transplanted liver. Dr Jorge Reyes, the surgeon who had performed the second transplant on Benito, only found out about his patient's decision six months after Benito stopped taking his drugs. When he did, he just couldn't accept that the fifteen-year-old knew best. 'When he left here he felt well,' says Reyes. 'He was totally independent and had very good liver function . . . Then, months later, we discover he's complaining of headaches and is not taking his medication and appears to have taken a conscious decision to terminate his life, claiming that the medication is making him suffer. As someone who takes care of children I see this as an emergency situation . . . but also that there is a very, very serious behavioural disorder here. Why would he decide to stop taking his medication if he was functioning normally?'

Benito knew exactly why. 'I don't want to die,' he said. 'But I'm tired of living in pain. I'd rather stay at home and live as close as I can to a natural life. I know what I'm doing. I'm not trying to commit suicide. But I don't want to live like that . . . I should have the right to make my own decision.'[15]

The gulf between Jorge Reyes, the medical practitioner, and Benito Agrelo, the transplant patient, could not have been wider. Benito believed he had a fundamental right to decide his future, even if that meant hastening his death. Reyes felt that the desire for death was a sign of abnormality. It was clear to him that Benito had to be saved from himself. 'To have an adolescent who does not want to take his medicine is very common,' he says. 'Many children have a hard time dealing with it but there are ways of helping them and rehabilitating them to make them feel like they are normal kids again. This was missed here in a terrible way because we could not get hold of the family.'

Reyes tried to keep in touch with the Agrelos, but they were so disillusioned with the treatments that they returned all his letters saying they didn't need his help any more. So Reyes had little or no communication with Benito. He was in Pittsburgh, while the Agrelos lived in Coral Springs, Florida. Despite this, the surgeon decided that the fifteen-year-old was not entitled to decide his future and asked Florida's Department of Health and Rehabilitative Services (HRS) to have him brought into hospital where he could be persuaded to take his medicines. The HRS, whose job is to protect children from abuse, decided that this was a case of parental neglect. It is hard not to conclude that what happened next amounted to an organized officially sanctioned kidnap. An HRS official arrived outside the Agrelos' Coral Springs home after dark on 8 June 1994 armed with an order to take Benito into protective custody and accompanied by an ambulance and three police officers. One of them was Sergeant Roy Dobson.

'It was really tumultuous,' he says. 'His mother was quite upset at the police. She was shouting that Benny wanted to die in peace . . . I had to stand and not let Benny back into the house. Benny was so upset that he actually punched a window out, but we could not let him go back into the house as we were frightened that there would be a barricade situation.'

Eventually the police persuaded Benito to walk towards the ambulance. Detective Charles Amos was also at the scene and remembers the moment: 'The entire Agrelo family was outside the house. When we got him to the back of the ambulance, Benny's brother was yelling the whole time and telling him to put up a fight and kick . . . Then his brother pushed me aggressively once or twice, still yelling and screaming. We did not want to fight with him – so we arrested him and put him in handcuffs and that's when Benny got irritated and decided he was not going to go in the back of the ambulance.'

Because Benito had no outward signs of injury, the ambulance driver was reluctant to take him in the vehicle and had to be instructed to do so by his supervisors. 'He [Benito] was very agitated and crying,' says Thomas Tropeano, one of the paramedics on duty that day. 'He was saying that he wanted to stay home and die. He screamed: "I do not want to go. Nobody can tell me what to do." When he was in the ambulance he was very violent and very aggressive. He was trying to kick and scratch . . . so we had to restrain Benny and tie him to the stretcher with towels and put a face mask on him to stop him biting us.'

Benito Agrelo had become a prisoner, a captive to society's fear of death. The HRS ambulance drove him to Miami where he was held in a room on the fifteenth floor of Jackson Memorial Hospital. Benito was very angry when he first arrived, and he gave the nursing staff a tough time. Nurse Debbie Weppler was on duty the morning after his forced admission. 'He was very withdrawn and wouldn't give much as far as answers,' she recalls. 'He was very cut and dry, you know: "Get out of my room. I don't want to be treated. Go away, I just want to die." '

Weppler tried to calm Benito's frayed nerves, and eventually persuaded him to talk about his feelings, but was unable to win his co-operation. He refused to permit the medical team to do a tissue biopsy and an ultrasound test to determine the condition of his liver. Later that day Andreas Tzakis visited Benito and told him that even if he did start taking his medicines again, the chances were that his second liver was too far gone and that he would need a third transplant to save his life. Benito wasn't interested. With his family around him, he continued to refuse all medical treatments and investigations.

'No matter how much you talked to him and tried to explain from our point of view,' says Nurse Weppler, 'he was set in his mind that he did not want to be re-transplanted, nor did he want to take any more medications . . . My concern was that I didn't really know if he understood what "end-stage liver disease" meant – how sick he could get. He could start bleeding and become confused and not really be aware of what was going on in his environment . . . But I really felt after talking with him for a couple of days that he knew what he wanted. He had made an intelligent choice. He had weighed all the factors and really come to a conclusion . . . Benny knew that he was going to die. He had a full understanding of that. He said that he had prepared himself. He knew that his life wasn't long for this world and he wanted to stay at home with his friends and family. And that was one of the reasons that he was so angry about being in the hospital.'

The Agrelos are Catholics who believe that everything in life has a purpose, even sickness and death. They were convinced that Benito was mature enough to decide his own future. Far from neglecting him, they insisted that love and compassion for the welfare of a sick child were behind their support of his actions. Doctors, they felt, had to respect patients' wishes, even if that meant they were taking decisions that would hasten their patients' death. Benito's mother, Armanda, decided to ask a judge to strike out the HRS detention order and tell Jackson Memorial Hospital to release Benito. The issue was heard by Broward County Circuit Judge Arthur Birkin. He visited the 'prisoner' in Jackson Memorial Hospital and listened to four hours of testimony from lawyers on both sides before quashing the order and freeing Benito. Birkin decided that he was not under pressure from his family and was old enough to take an informed decision.

Three days after his capture, on 11 June 1994, Benito went home to spend his last days in peace with his family. He had little time left: without medication for eight months, his body's immune system had seriously damaged his transplanted liver. Slowly, it became less efficient at removing the toxins from his body. His abdomen swelled. He lost the vitality that had transformed his body when he first stopped taking the anti-rejection drugs. He ate erratically, vomited frequently and his eyes became so sensitive to light that he was forced to live in a darkened room lit only by the light of the TV screen that took his imagination to the places his ailing body could no longer visit. He never had second thoughts. 'I made my decision and they weren't going to change my mind,' he said, a few weeks after his release from hospital. 'I was tired of being a guinea pig. Why be afraid of dying? It's pain – living with pain – that's hard. No more doctors. No more operations. No more transplants. I don't want to live like that any more.'[16]

Benito's story touched a sympathetic nerve in the nation. The Agrelos were deluged with letters, cards, gifts and phone calls after the court hearing, many from well-wishers who had faced a death in their families and wanted Benito to know he had their full support. 'You have made the most difficult decision a person can make,' wrote one woman whose son, Nicky, had died eight years earlier. 'I know because I had to make that choice for Nicky. He was tired of hurting too. Take care and give Nicky a hug when you see him.'[17]

By the middle of August, it was clear that Benito was dying. He had stopped eating and was drifting in and out of a coma. When he was conscious, he lay in bed covered with wet towels to reduce his temperature, unable to do more than stare at his fish tank. His family and friends took it in turns to sleep on the floor. Claudine Com took time off work to stay close to Benito during these closing days. On the last night of his life she kept vigil by his bedside with his sister Ava. 'It was Friday night,' she recalls. 'He'd been bleeding all day long from his nose and mouth and we just kept changing the towels and washing him down. His breathing had become very, very deep and very laboured. And every so often it would stop for a few seconds and we'd all kind of panic. And then his very laboured breathing would start again. He wasn't really coherent at all. We just tried to keep him as comfortable as possible. As the night wore on, I guess exhaustion took over at that point and she and I both slept. His mum woke us up very softly and told us that he had just passed away. Just before he had, he'd kind of opened his eyes, looked at her and held out his arms and said: "Oh, God," and then he just collapsed on her. It was very peaceful. We were in his room. The only sound we could hear at that point was the bubbles from the aquarium. We were just all together. There were no outsiders. There was no one to make us feel uncomfortable. We could be at ease with him.'

Benito Agrelo died on 20 August 1994.[18] The teenage boy whose life had been so unbearable had won his last battle. He had argued that the quality of life is ultimately more important than its length and, in so doing, cast an uncomfortable light on the philosophy that underpins our late-twentieth-century medical systems. Benito was on the verge of adulthood, and doctors could not force an adult to take medicines against their will. So, was Benito's disturbing story an exception, or does it raise deeper questions about the direction in which transplant surgery is driving medical practice? Is the power of the technology preventing doctors from seeing that sometimes it is more humane to advise against further treatment than endlessly to prolong suffering in the vain hope of a cure? The balance is undoubtedly hard to find. But the short lives of Benito Agrelo and Laura Davies seem to show that the scales are tipping in favour of unnecessary medical intervention.

'The trouble is,' says Dr Moneim Fadali, the cardiac surgeon from Los Angeles, 'that we are so petrified and afraid of death that we just run away, and in escaping from death we seek to extend our lives, no matter what. . . . You cannot separate science from ethics. You cannot do simply what it is possible to do. You have to do what is right.'

Postscript
The Mystery of Betty's Body

In the late 1960s the English transplant surgeon Roy [now Sir Roy] Calne made a remarkable observation. He conducted a series of fifty-five experimental liver transplants on pigs, without giving the animals treatment to prevent rejection, expecting them to reject their new livers and die within a few weeks. Most did. But some of the animals survived and went on to live long, healthy lives, their new livers working perfectly for up to five years. One survived drug-free for eleven years. This seemed to defy the laws of immunology.

'The results here cannot be explained in terms of close relationship of donor and recipient,' Calne reported in the *British Medical Journal*[1] '. . . the transplanted liver can be accepted even when the donor and recipient are from widely disparate genetic sources – that is, different porcine breeds. . . . If the mechanism of acceptance were discovered, clinical application might resolve many of the present difficulties of organ transplantation.'

It was a tantalizing but baffling observation. By some unknown process, the bodies of the surviving pigs seemed to accept their transplanted livers as if they were their own. Under the microscope, the liver cells showed little or no evidence of rejection. This even held true for the livers of those pigs that died early deaths: they had succumbed to other complications. The prestigious medical journal the *Lancet* neatly summed up feelings about Calne's drug-free survivors when it commented on the work in an editorial entitled: 'Strange English Pigs'.

Calne's pigs threw a rather large spanner into the works of the theory of immunology. Until then, there had been only one way of making the body accept a transplanted organ without using lethal X-rays or toxic chemicals: the Trojan Horse approach discovered by the zoologist Peter Medawar in the early 1950s.[2]

Medawar's technique worked and was free of side effects, but it could never have been a practical method of avoiding rejection in transplanted patients because it involved injecting unborn or newly born animals. But if a pig could accept a transplanted liver with no anti-rejection treatment, surely it might be possible to find a way of making a person's body do the same. Perhaps the body might be persuaded to tolerate other organs as well? If doctors could unravel the mystery of Calne's 'Strange English Pigs', they would be on the threshold of finding the Holy Grail of spare-part surgery: a means of preventing rejection with no unwanted side effects.

Calne took his experiment a step further to find out if the 'liver effect' was peculiar to the pig or if tolerance could be induced in other species. He performed another series of liver transplants and found that some rats accepted transplanted livers without drug treatment. But what about humans? He couldn't just refuse to treat a group of transplanted patients with immuno-suppressive drugs. If he did that, he would be struck off the medical register for unethical behaviour. Yet that was the only way of discovering if humans could become tolerant to transplanted livers. It looked as if the question would never be answered – until Betty Baird rang her doctor in Denver, Colorado, in 1981 to tell him that she had flushed her anti-rejection medicines down the toilet and was never going to take any more.

Betty Baird had a liver transplant in 1979. It saved her life but, as we saw in Chapter 5,[3] the physical and psychological side effects of the drugs she needed to stay alive were crippling. Eventually she had reached the same conclusion as Benito Agrelo: that she would rather have a few months of good-quality life than an eternity of distressing side effects. 'I just decided one day that I was not going to take the medicine any more,' says Betty. 'I didn't care if it killed me. I just decided I don't like myself like this. So I walked to the bathroom, took them all out of the medicine cabinet, popped the tops off and flushed them away. I remember sitting there, just watching them and crying.'

About a month later she plucked up the courage to tell her

doctor. 'At first they didn't believe me,' she says. 'My doctor was furious. He just kept telling me I was going to die: "You cannot live without the medicine. You can't just quit it." He wanted me to go back on it and he'd cut it down a little. I told him: "No. I'm doing fine without it . . . I feel a lot better. I know I'm doing better without it." They kept wanting me to come down for more tests . . . So long as I was feeling good I didn't go . . . You just kind of know your own body. If I'd have been sick or having pains or anything, I'm sure I would have gone right back and got on [the drugs] . . . It was just a gut feeling.'

Unlike Benito Agrelo's body, Betty's did not reject her new liver. Since she stopped taking her medicine in June 1981 she has remained in good health. There is now a handful of these living enigmas: transplant patients who have thrown away their drugs and who, like Betty, have not lost their organs or their lives. Most of these survivors have had new livers. A few have been given a kidney.[4] The understandable concern expressed by their doctors in the early days eventually turned into curiosity when they realized that inside the bodies of these drug-free patients, they might find the key to the future of transplant surgery.

'As the years went on we stopped trying to force or intimidate them to go back onto drugs,' says Tom Starzl, the surgeon who gave Betty her new liver. 'But more important than that, we began to think that there has to be a secret here explaining why these grafts had been accepted that could help all other patients.'

Medical researchers in several countries are now doing their best to unravel the mystery. In 1992 Tom Starzl invited a number of these drug-free transplant patients to come to the University of Pittsburgh and undergo a series of tests. His research team took samples of their transplanted organs and other parts of their bodies and inspected them under a microscope. Starzl says his colleagues were astonished by what they found. The body tissues of all the transplant patients who had come off their medicines had undergone a fundamental change. They were no longer the people they had been when they were born. They had become biological chimeras: their bodies had transformed into a mixture of two different individuals. Certain mobile cells from the transplanted livers had migrated to many parts of each recipient's body and were co-existing happily alongside their own cells.

The process had also worked in reverse: similar cells from the recipient had travelled to and were living inside each transplanted liver. This seemed to run counter to the known laws of immunology – after all, transplant surgery's biggest problem has been the body's tendency to destroy any foreign object in its midst. Yet here were people living happily and healthily, not just with a transplanted organ inside them but with foreign cells co-existing with their own.

'Once the cells get out,' says Tom Starzl, 'and get a foothold like Columbus arriving in America, it's pretty hard to uproot them. And those are the cells that are inducing acceptance of that kidney or of that liver.'

Starzl believes some degree of cell migration takes place with all successful transplantation, irrespective of the organ. It is most noticeable with the liver because this organ has its own mini-immune system, with a large number of mobile cells. His theory is that, straight after an organ transplant, a conflict develops in the body. Not only do cells from the recipient's immune system try to attack and destroy the transplant but cells from the donor organ itself attack the body.[5] There are two possible outcomes to this struggle: either the transplant is overwhelmed and destroyed or a balance is reached in which the warring cells appear to declare a truce and cease fighting. In pigs, the armistice can come about naturally. In humans, it seems to require a temporary period of anti-rejection treatment to keep the warring parties apart long enough for peace to be declared.

There are many unanswered questions about the importance of cell migration. Medical researchers are divided as to whether it causes tolerance or is itself the effect of another still-unknown process that makes the body accept a transplanted liver. They do not understand why such a relatively small number of cells from a transplant can have such a profound effect on the huge army lined up against them in the recipient's body. Neither do they know why, in some people, the warring cells declare a truce that spares the transplant while in others they fight to the finish. But transplant immunologists have already produced tolerance in laboratory animals. Sir Roy Calne has now persuaded pigs' bodies to accept a transplanted kidney indefinitely, without the need for long-term anti-rejection treatment, by giving the animals a few large doses of Cyclosporin immediately after the transplant and then stopping all drug treatment, which seems to create the conditions necessary for successful cell migration and therefore for tolerance.

'This is a type of approach that could be used in the clinic,' says Sir Roy. 'What we are hoping to do is make the recipients' immune system inactive for a short period of time while the graft is put in place and while it becomes "imprinted" with the characteristics of the transplant. Then when we stop the drug treatment, the body won't see it as foreign. That's the concept. It may be that it is much too simple an explanation, but that's how we see it and it seems to work. It's a positive experiment.'

Transplant surgery could be on the verge of a discovery of fundamental importance, one that would change the way we think about the human body in just as radical a way as did the first successful organ transplant. Without the need for risky drug treatments to prevent rejection, the question we might soon be facing is not how do we do it, but how much of it should we do.

'Oh, I think it would completely transform attitudes,' says Sir Roy Calne. 'We would then be prepared to transplant organs that we are not transplanting at the moment – such as limbs, endocrine glands, even gonads, the testis and ovary, which would produce great excitement in the media. I think that skin transplants might even then be possible . . . So it's been our goal – it's the Holy Grail of transplantation.'

Appendix
Transplant Survival Records to end of 1994

Statistics from UCLA Tissue Typing Laboratory

(items marked* from Addenbrooke's Hospital, Cambridge)

	Date of transplant	Years since transplant	Initials	Age at transplant	Age now	Location
HEART						
Longest	9/6/73	21 yrs 6 m	R.E.	48	69	Foch Hospital, Paris, France
Longest child	1/11/84	10 yrs 1 m	S.R.	9 months	10 yrs	Texas Heart Institute, Houston, USA
Youngest	16/10/87	7 yrs 2 m	P.H.	3 hours	7 yrs	Loma Linda Uni, California, USA
Oldest	20/11/90	4 yrs 1 m	W.H.	73	77	Heart Centre, N. Rhine Westphalia, Germany
KIDNEY						
Longest: Living Related Donor	31/1/63	31 yrs 11 m	R.P.	38	69	Uni of Colorado, Denver, USA
Longest: Living Unrelated Donor	5/7/79	15 yrs 5 m	H.L.	33	48	Yonsel Uni, Korea
Longest: Cadaveric Donor	10/10/64	30 yrs 2 m	Y.T.	31	61	Necker Hospital, Paris, France
Longest: No Drug Treatment – Living Related Donor	9/2/63	31 yrs 10 m	K.P.	21	52	Uni of Colorado, Denver, USA
Youngest: Living Related Donor	17/4/68	26 yrs 8 m	D.H.	1 day	26	Children's Hospital, Cincinnati, USA

	Date of transplant	Years since transplant	Initials	Age at transplant	Age now	Location
LIVER						
Longest: Cadaveric Donor	22/1/70	24 yrs 11 m	K.H.	3	27	Uni of Colorado, Denver, USA
Longest: Living Related donor – partial transplant	27/11/89	5 yrs 1 m	A.S.	1 yr	6 yrs	Uni of Chicago, USA
Oldest	11/8/86	8 yrs	S.M.	76	84	Uni of Pittsburgh, USA
Youngest	12/6/92	2 yrs 6 m	D.E.	12 days	2 yrs	Uni of Chicago, USA
LUNG						
Longest: Single	1/1/85	9 yrs 11 m	J.H.	45	54	Toronto General Hospital, Canada
Youngest: Single	27/10/91	2 yrs 2 m	J.R.	17 days	2 yrs	Stanford University, California, USA
Oldest: Single	9/1/93	1 yr 11 m	E.S.	68	69	N. Indiana Heart Institute, USA
Longest: Double	26/11/86	8 yrs 1 m	A.H.	42	50	Toronto General Hospital, Canada
Youngest: Double	21/6/94	6 m	M.C.	2 m	8 m	Washington Uni, St Louis, USA
Oldest: Double	26/8/93	1 yr 4 m	K.M.	62	63	Uni of Pittsburgh, USA

	Date of transplant	Years since transplant	Initials	Age at transplant	Age now	Location
PANCREAS						
Longest	25/7/78	16 yrs 5 m	M.W.	31	47	Uni of Minnesota, Minneapolis, USA
SMALL BOWEL						
Longest: Cadaveric Donor	18/3/89	5 yrs 9 m	Anon.	5 m	6 yrs	Necker Hospital, Paris, France
MULTIVISCERAL						
Longest	14/10/91	3 yrs 2 m	P.B.	32	35	Uni of Pittsburgh, USA
Most Organs (6)*	15/3/94	7 m	S.H.	32	32	Addenbrooke's Hospital, Cambridge, UK

	Date of transplant	Years since transplant	Initials	Age at transplant	Age now	Location
Heart and Bone Marrow						
Longest	22/3/94	9 months	J.T.	50	50	Uni of Pittsburgh, USA
Heart and Lung						
Longest	5/11/82	12 yrs 1m	R.G.	40	52	Stanford University, California, USA
Youngest	14/6/89	5 yrs 6m	M.M.	4 m	5 yrs	Stanford University, California, USA
Oldest	16/12/89	5 yrs	Anon	67	72	St Antonius Hospital, Nieuwegein, Netherlands
Heart, Lungs and Liver						
Longest*	17/12/86	8 yrs	D.T.	35	43	Papworth and Addenbrooke's Hospitals, Cambridge, UK
Kidney and Bone Marrow						
Longest	14/12/92	2 yrs	S.M.	50	52	Uni of Pittsburgh, USA
Liver and Bone Marrow						
Longest	7/6/92	2 yrs 6 m	J.S.	31	33	Uni of Pittsburgh, USA
Liver and Heart						
Longest	7/7/92	2 yrs 6 m	R.F.	47	49	Mayo Clinic, Minnesota, USA

	Date of transplant	Years since transplant	Initials	Age at transplant	Age now	Location
Liver and Kidney						
Longest	28/12/83	11 yrs	J.M.	27	38	University Hospital, Innsbruck, Austria
Youngest	16/5/94	7 m	B.C.	7 m	14 m	Edouard Heriot Hospital, Lyon, France
Liver and Pancreas						
Longest	1/7/88	6 yrs	A.B.	39	45	Uni of Pittsburgh, USA
Liver and Pancreatic Islets						
Longest	16/3/90	4 yrs	F.S.	52	56	Uni of Pittsburgh, USA
Liver, Pancreatic Islets & Bone Marrow – Longest	15/3/90	3 yrs	K.L.	24	27	Essen Uni Medical School, Germany
Liver and Single Lung						
Longest	4/5/90	4 yrs	M.W.	50	54	Uni of Toronto, Canada
Liver and Small Bowel						
Longest	24/7/90	4 yrs	T.G.	3	7	Uni of Pittsburgh, USA
Pancreas and Kidney						
Longest: Cadaveric Donor	10/4/81	13 yrs 8m	A.M.	31	44	Uni Hospital, Zurich, Switzerland

Notes

1. Dogs' Legs, Cats' Kidneys and Monkey Glands

1. Reported in Charles C. Thomas, *Alexis Carrel – Visionary Surgeon*, p. 29.
2. The first person to attempt to transplant a kidney was Dr Emerich Ullman, an Austrian surgeon, who grafted a dog's kidney into the neck of the same animal. A Viennese medical journal published the results of his work on 24 January 1902. In the same paper, Ullman also discussed two previous kidney transplants he had done: from one dog to another and from a dog to a goat. He claimed some success with these experiments but abandoned transplantation after this. Carrel knew of Ullman's work and refers to it in some of his papers.
3. Alexis Carrel, 'Transplantation in Mass of the Kidneys', 1908, *Journal of Experimental Medicine*, p. 98.
4. Alexis Carrel, letter to Theodor Kocher, 9 May 1914, quoted in *Surgery and Life* by Theodore Malinin, p. 49.
5. Walter R. Howden, in the *Abolitionist*, as quoted in *Surgery and Life* by Theodore Malinin, p. 50.
6. René Kuss and Pierre Bourget, *An Illustrated History of Organ Transplantation*, p. 29.
7. Theodore Malinin, *Surgery and Life*, p. 51.
8. Samuel Pozzi, as quoted in René Kuss and Pierre Bourget, *An Illustrated History of Organ Transplantation*, p. 30.
9. The technical term for joining blood vessels together.
10. Karolinska Institute citation, 1912. Nobel Prize in Medicine.
11. The function of testosterone is to control the development of secondary sexual characteristics.
12. Sydney B. Flower, *The Life of a Man: a Biography of John R. Brinkley*.
13. David Hamilton, *The Monkey Gland Affair*, p. 34.

14. S. Voronoff and E. Retterer, 'Structure of the Chimpanzee Testicle and Physiological Effects of its Transplantation', 1923. Quoted in David Hamilton's *The Monkey Gland Affair*, p. 57.

15. *New York Times*, 19 June 1922.

16. 1926 Congress of the French Association for the Advancement of Science.

17. 1927 in Budapest. Quoted in David Hamilton's *The Monkey Gland Affair*, p. 101.

18. David Hamilton, *The Monkey Gland Affair*, p. 72.

19. Ibid., p. 135.

20. Ibid.

21. Ibid., p. 141.

22. Mathieu Jaboulay, 'Kidney Grafts in the Antecubital Fossa by Arterial and Venous Anastomosis', *Lyon Medical*, 1906, 107:575.

23. Ernest Unger, 'Kidney Transplantation', 1910, translated from German by Ronald G. Landes.

24. Ibid.

25. Harold Neuhof, 'Transplantation of Tissues', p. 263.

26. Yu Yu Voronoy, 'Blocking the reticulo-endothelial system in man in some forms of mercuric chloride intoxication and the transplantation of the cadaver kidney as a method of treatment for the aneuria resulting from the intoxication', *Siglo Medico*, 1937, 97:296.

27. Voronoy had transplanted a kidney from an O blood group donor into a B group recipient. This is now regarded as an incompatibility that will usually provoke a fierce form of rejection.

28. See note 26.

29. In 1947, three American surgeons, David Hume, Charles Hufnagel, and Ernest Landsteiner, transplanted a cadaver kidney into the arm of a critically ill patient at the Peter Bent Brigham Hospital in Boston. The patient, a woman, was in a deep coma. Her own kidneys had failed ten days earlier, following an illegal abortion, and she seemed certain to die. The hospital did not yet have an artificial kidney and, in desperation, her doctors decided to give her a temporary transplant believing that her own kidneys might recover if they could keep her alive for a few more days. The plan worked. A kidney taken from an accident victim and transplanted into the patient produced urine for twenty-four hours. It was removed two

days later when the woman's own kidneys began to recover. See Dr Hufnagel's account of this operation in Francis D. Moore's *Transplant: the Give and Take of Tissue Transplantation*, pp. 40–41.

30. Sir Peter Medawar, *Memoir of a Thinking Radish*, pp. 76–7.

31. Ibid., p. 80.

32. Medawar calls these 'pinch grafts' – small buttons of skin about the size of an eight-year-old's fingernail cut by lifting the skin with a hook and slicing it off with a scalpel.

33. T. Gibson and P. Medawar, 'The Fate of Skin Homografts in Man', *Journal of Anatomy*, London, 1943, pp. 299–310.

2. Hard Graft

1. Lawler, Richard H., 'Medicine's Living History: Dr Richard Lawler recalls the first successful kidney transplant', *Medical World News*, 14 April 1972, p. 52.

2. Ibid.

3. Ibid., p. 54.

4. Ibid., p. 56.

5. *New York Times*, 20 June 1950.

6. *Time* magazine, 3 July 1950.

7. *Newsweek*, 3 July 1950.

8. Ibid., p. 56.

9. Lawler, Richard H., *et al.*, 'Homotransplantation of the Kidney in the Human – Supplemental Report of a Case', *Journal of the American Medical Association*, 1 September 1951, vol. 147, pp. 45, 46.

10. American Urological Association public relations committee statement. Quoted in the *Chicago Daily News*, 22 May 1951.

11. Ibid., p. 57.

12. The Peter Bent Brigham Hospital has since been renamed the Brigham and Women's Hospital.

13. An illness commonly called 'water on the brain', which causes a dangerous rise in pressure inside the skull. It was treated in the 1950s by conducting excess fluid around the brain via a tube into one of the patient's ureters, so that it was excreted into the bladder.

This operation necessitated the removal of one of the kidneys, which surgeons were then able to transplant into another patient.

14. René Kuss says this attitude began to change in the mid 1960s when kidney transplantation ceased to be a highly experimental treatment and began to save patients' lives.

15. *The Courage to Fail*, BBC1, 23 November 1987.

16. It came from a thirty-four-year-old woman with an irreparably damaged ureter, preventing urine from passing into her bladder.

17. One patient lived for twenty days; one died on the operating table; one survived thanks to a recovery in the patient's remaining kidney. The transplant itself began to stop functioning after thirty days. The fifth and last in the series done in April 1951 was taken from a guillotined prisoner. 'We had to go there,' he told the author, 'perform the extremely painful act of cutting open the decapitated man, rapidly extracting his kidneys and carrying them back to the hospital as rapidly as possible where the recipient was on the operating table waiting for his or her new kidney . . . Personally I never had the courage to go myself, so I sent my assistant who was younger and perhaps more courageous than I and who accepted such a difficult task.' This transplant was removed after forty-eight hours. See R. Kuss, J. Teinturier and P. Millez's paper, 'Some Experiments on Renal Grafting In Man', published in *Mémoires de L'Academie de Chirurgie*, 1951, 77:755.

18. Accounts of this transplant are given in René Kuss's *An Illustrated History of Organ Transplantation*', pp. 43–44, and in an article by Jean Hamburger published in *History of Transplantation: 35 Recollections*, edited by Paul Terasaki, p. 63.

19. The artificial kidney machine was invented during the war by Wilhelm Kolff. It was developed into a practical therapeutic tool at the Peter Bent Brigham Hospital where it began to be used in 1947 and 1948 to tide over patients suffering from a temporary failure of their kidneys. The early machines were not sophisticated enough to keep dying patients alive indefinitely. Problems with the attachment of the machine to the patient's blood vessels meant that it could only be used a few times until the end of the 1950s when a better system was devised. Prior to this, the use of the artificial kidney on patients with irreversible kidney failure was discouraged. Instead, it

was used to keep patients awaiting a transplant in a sufficiently good condition to survive the rigours of surgery. 'I think it's reasonable to say that without this thing transplantation never would have got started,' Dr John P. Merrill, the Head of Nephrology at the Peter Bent Brigham Hospital in this period, commented in a TV documentary *The Transplanters*.

20. D.M. Hume, J.P. Merrill, B.J. Miller and G.W. Thorn, 'Experiences with Renal Homotransplantation in the Human: Report of Nine Cases', *Journal of Clinical Investigation*, February 1955, vol. 34.

21. The correct medical name for Bright's disease is glomerulo-nephritis, an inflammation of the kidney (nephron) that begins in the small collecting devices (glomeruli) that filter the blood.

22. Hume wrote that there was a 'severe degree' of blocking of the arteries in the transplanted kidney – one sign of rejection, but he found no evidence of 'thrombosis, infarction, calcification, infection or glomerulonephritis' in the organ. See Hume's paper 'Experience with Renal Homotransplantation in the Human: Report of Nine Cases', *Journal of Clinical Investigation*, February 1955, vol. 34, pp. 366–367.

23. A homotransplant was then the technical term for the transplantation of tissue or organs from one animal to another of the same species. It is now called an allotransplant.

24. D.M. Hume, J.P. Merrill, B.J. Miller and G.W. Thorn, 'Experiences with Renal Homotransplantation', p. 377.

25. Hume left the hospital to take up a post at the Naval Medical Research Institute in Bethesda, Maryland.

26. Murray had done six transplants after David Hume left the Peter Bent Brigham Hospital in 1953.

27. Francis D. Moore, *A Miracle and a Privilege: Recounting a Half Century of Surgical Advance*, p. 173.

28. Francis D. Moore, *Transplant. The Give and Take of Tissue Transplantation*, pp. 101–102.

29. Peter Medawar, *Memoir of a Thinking Radish*, p. 111.

30. The placenta is the cord that unites the unborn animal to its mother while it is in the womb. It provides the baby calf with oxygen and food and removes waste products.

31. Peter Medawar, *Memoir of a Thinking Radish*, p. 132.

32. Ibid., p. 134.

33. See p. 110 of Francis D. Moore's *Transplant: The Give and Take of Tissue Transplantation*. Sometimes the dose of X-rays was designed only to weaken the attacking cells, not destroy them totally. Then the bone marrow transfusion was omitted.

34. She received 600 roentgens. Only one other transplant patient treated with X-rays in Boston received such a high dose. Most received doses ranging from 200 to 400 roentgens, enough to weaken but not kill the cells responsible for rejection.

35. He planned to do twelve but complications forced him to abandon two of the planned transplants. See the paper 'Kidney Transplantation in Modified Recipients' by J.E. Murray, J.P. Merrill *et al.*, published in *Annals of Surgery*, 1962, 156:337.

36. See the paper 'Homologous Human Kidney Transplantation' by R. Kuss, M.D. Legrain *et al.*, published in 1962 in the *Postgraduate Medical Journal*, vol. 38, pp. 528–536.

37. The sixth patient transplanted with a kidney in Hamburger's series lived for almost two years after X-ray irradiation.

38. 'Kidney Transplantation in Modified Recipients' op. cit.

39. See pages 2 and 3.

40. Quoted from the paper 'Three Clinical Cases of Renal Transplantation' by J. Hopewell, B.Y. Calne and I. Beswick, *British Medical Journal*, 15 February 1964.

41. 6-mercaptopurine was first synthesized in 1952 by George Hitchings and Gertrude Elion of the Burroughs Wellcome Company. They were looking for drugs active against leukaemia but suspected that 6-MP might have immuno-suppressive effects. Hitchings and Elion eventually won the Nobel Prize for this and other related work.

42. Robert Schwartz and William Damashek, two haematologists working at Tuft's University in Boston, had tested 6-MP for immuno-suppressive properties. The results of their work were first published in 1958 in the Proceedings of the Society for Experimental Biology & Medicine (vol. 99, pp. 164–167) and later republished in *Nature* (June 1959, vol. 183, p. 1682) with the title 'Drug Induced Immunologic Tolerance'. Schwartz and Damashek tested the drug on rabbits and found that it prolonged the survival

of skin grafts. Kendrick Porter, a pathologist from St Mary's Hospital, London, heard of Schwartz and Damashek's work when they presented it at a conference in London in September 1959, and then told Sir Roy Calne.

43. The experiments were done from autumn 1959 until January 1960 and the results were published in the *Lancet* (20 February 1960, pp. 417–418). Kidneys transplanted into dogs not given the drug usually ceased to function after four to eight days. The longest lived survivor in those animals given 6-MP were twenty-one and forty-seven days. Charles Zukoski and David Hume, of the Medical College of Virginia, were also testing the drug on dogs at this time. They had animals living for up to thirty-four days with 6-MP. Their results were published a few months after Calne's.

44. Before leaving for America, he tried giving 6-MP to three kidney transplant patients, the first clinical use of the substance. They all failed, the patients dying three days, eleven days and forty-nine days after their operations. Sir Roy believes they were all too sick to benefit from a transplant because he did not then have the expertise with the artificial kidney to be able to improve their condition enough to survive the rigours of a transplant operation. See J. Hopewell, R.Y. Calne and I. Beswick, 'Three Clinical Cases of Renal Transplantation', 1964, *British Medical Journal*.

45. Its full chemical name is azathioprine.

46. 'Homologous Human Kidney Transplantation', op. cit. pp. 528–531.

47. The kidney was rejected in January 1964 and replaced with a second transplant. The patient died nearly six months later. See the paper by J.P. Merrill, J.E. Murray *et al.*, 'Successful Transplantation of Kidney from Human Cadaver' published in *Journal of the American Medical Association*, 3 August 1963, vol. 185, pp. 347–353. Also, the paper by J.E. Murray, R.E. Wilson *et al.*, 'Five Years' Experience with Renal Transplantation with Immunosuppressive Drugs' in *Annals of Surgery*, July–December 1968, vol. 168, pp. 416–433.

48. Willard E. Goodwin & Donald Martin, quoted in Tom Starzl's *The Puzzle People: Memoirs of a Transplant Surgeon*, p. 110.

49. Tom Starzl, *The Puzzle People: Memoirs of a Transplant Surgeon*, p. 109.

50. Eight of the first ten patients in this series were still alive at the time of the meeting. They had survived from between 46 and 218 days. See Starzl, Marchioro and Waddell's paper 'The Reversal of Rejection in Human Renal Homografts with Subsequent Development of Homograft Tolerance' in *Surgery, Gynaecology & Obstetrics*, October 1963, vol. 117, pp. 385–395. Subsequently, six of those eight patients went on to live for more than twenty-five years on their transplanted kidneys. Five were still alive in November 1995.

51. Tom Starzl, *The Puzzle People: Memoirs of a Transplant Surgeon*, p. 110.

52. Starzl's 'double drug' therapy was partly inspired by work done in Los Angeles by Willard E. Goodwin at UCLA, who'd first noticed the dramatic ability of high-dosage steroids to reverse acute rejection. Starzl also gave his patients a third drug called Actinomycin C, but says this was not as significant against rejection as Prednisone.

53. T.E. Starzl, T.L. Marchioro and W.R. Waddell, op. cit. p. 392. Starzl has told the author that he gave his patients up to 200 mg of Prednisone a day, a dose that in 1963 was considered 'astronomical'.

54. Quoted in *History of Transplantation: 35 Recollections* edited by Paul Terasaki, p. 67.

55. Before the transplant, Yvette Thibault's thymus gland was irradiated, her spleen was removed and she was given Imuran to prevent rejection. Since then she has been given a mixture of Imuran and cortisone. She is currently only taking a low dose of cortisone.

56. Two surgeons shared the $700,000 award: the other was Dr E. Donnall Thomas of the Fred Hutchinson Cancer Research Centre in Seattle. He was honoured for pioneering the use of methotrexate to make bone-marrow transplants a reality.

57. Reuters report, 'Nobel Prize Winner Says He Thought He Was Dreaming', 8 October 1990.

58. Citation, Nobel Prize for Medicine, 1990.

59. *Le Monde*, 10 October 1990.

60. *Le Quotidien du Medicine*, 10 October 1990.

61. 'The First Successful Organ Transplants In Man' delivered by Joseph Murray on 8 December 1990.

62. See page 47. Murray has told the author that he did know about Kuss's successes. However, he says he didn't regard them as significant, as the French transplant team used X-rays in combination with 6-MP to save the two patients' lives while he had used drug therapy alone in his 1962 success. For Murray, then, any use of unpredictable X-rays disqualified Kuss from claiming a 'world first' – even though the French surgeon's first patient lived for nearly a year and a half on a kidney taken from an unrelated person. In the circumstances it was, perhaps, not the wisest of judgements.

63. 31 October 1990, letter to Professor Tom Starzl, University of Pittsburgh.

64. Hamburger died in 1992.

65. Tom Starzl, *The Puzzle People*, p. 105.

3. The Man with the Golden Hands

1. Quoted in *One Life*, Christiaan Barnard and Curtis Bill Pepper, p. 367.

2. Ibid.

3. Ibid.

4. Ibid., p. 369.

5. Christiaan Barnard, *The Second Life*, pp. 11–12.

6. By then Hume had left military service and returned to civilian life.

7. Quotes from Christiaan Barnard and Curtis Bill Pepper, *One Life*, pp. 336–337.

8. Ibid., p. 347.

9. Edward Darvall, ibid., p. 374.

10. Quoted in *One Life*, Christiaan Barnard and Curtis Bill Pepper, p. 375.

11. Ibid.

12. *One Life*, Christiaan Barnard and Curtis Bill Pepper, p. 401.

13. 'Tributes Pour in from Abroad', *Cape Times*, 6 December 1967.

4. The Knife-edge of Survival

1. Quoted in *One Life* by Christiaan Barnard and Bill Curtis Pepper, p. 457.
2. Ibid.
3. They increased the amount of Prednisone, the anti-inflammatory steroid.
4. The lung infection that killed Louis Washkansky was caused by a bacterium called *pseudomonas aeruginosa*.
5. The 'Great Karoo' is the large semi-desert area surrounding the town of Beaufort West, about 350 miles from Cape Town, in which Barnard grew up.
6. Christiaan Barnard, *The Second Life*, p. 131.
7. Ibid., p. 79.
8. Statistics taken from T. Thompson, *Hearts: Debakey and Cooley, Surgeons Extraordinary*.
9. The surgeon was Donald Ross. Donald Longmore was the patient's physician.
10. 18 June 1968.
11. 23 June 1968.
12. *Daily Telegraph*, 1 July 1968.
13. One transplant was done at Harefield Hospital, near London, in September 1973 by the heart surgeon Sir Magdi Yacoub. The patient, a 56-year-old man, lived just four hours. The next one wasn't done until 1979, when Sir Terence English began a series of heart transplants at Papworth Hospital in Cambridge.
14. He did eighteen but one was a re-transplant. Everett Thomas was given a second transplanted heart when his first was rejected after seven months. He died three days later.
15. Cooley restarted heart transplantation in 1982 with the introduction of a new drug treatment that greatly improved survival times.
16. Richard Lower had worked closely with Norman Shumway at Stanford Medical Centre in the early experimental period of heart transplant surgery. Most of the research papers were jointly authored by the two men. In 1965 Lower left Stanford to take up a job at the Medical College of Virginia.

17. *Black's Law Dictionary*, 4th edition, 1968, p. 488.
18. *New York Herald Tribune*, 27 May 1972.
19. Ibid.
20. Joseph Klett, Lower's first heart transplant patient, died seven days after receiving Bruce Tucker's heart. 'The reason was,' says Lower, 'that we did not, I think, at that time understand that we had to use a higher dosage of drugs to prevent rejection. We used the protocol that was being used in the kidney transplant patients and we didn't appreciate the fact that . . . heart transplant patients needed higher doses.' Richard Lower went on to do four heart transplants in 1968. Three died within days or weeks of their operation. Only one survived for an appreciable length of time: Louis Russell, transplanted in August 1968, lived for just over six years with his new heart.
21. In 1985 Dr Yuji Iwasaki of Tsukuba University transplanted a pancreas and a liver taken from two brain-dead patients and found himself facing charges of murder, manslaughter and corpse defilement. He was later cleared of all charges. Only five other surgeons in Japan had been prepared to risk taking organs from beating-heart cadavers, and all found themselves investigated for murder. No case has yet reached the courts.
22. A bill to legalize brain death was presented to the Diet, the lower house of the Japanese parliament in April 1994 but has made little progress. Discussion has been shelved on six occasions. It is now (December 1995) being debated by a parliamentary committee and will eventually be decided by a free vote of individual Diet members.
23. One reason for his survival might have been the addition of ALG (anti-lymphocyte globulin) to the drug treatment that Blaiberg received to prevent rejection. Tom Starzl, the liver transplant surgeon, had published an account of his clinical experience with ALG in January 1967, eleven months before Barnard's first heart transplant. Barnard did not use the serum on Louis Washkansky, but introduced it for his subsequent heart transplant patients, using it in combination with Imuran and Prednisone.
24. Dr Philip Blaiberg, *Looking at my Heart*, p. 97.
25. Statistics taken from T. Thompson, *Hearts: Debakery and Cooley, Surgeons Extraordinary*.

26. Statistics from Stanford University School of Medicine.

5. The Holy Grail

1. Its correct chemical name is azathioprine.
2. A hormone secreted by the adrenal glands but which can be made artificially as a pure chemical.
3. Tissue groups and blood groups are similar concepts. They mean that the tissue or blood cells contain various proteins, called antigens, which, when transplanted into another person, will be recognized by the body as 'foreign' and will, therefore, elicit an immune response. Red blood cells contain several that are important in blood transfusions (for example, the A, B, O, and Rh antigens). Human tissues are now thought to contain about seventy different antigens in three different positions, known as 'loci', on the surface of cells. These are identified as the A, the B and the DR loci. In 1970 only eleven antigens located on the A and B loci were known. The human tissue-typing system is known as the human leukocyte antigen (HLA) system.
4. In the mid-1930s, a British pathologist, Peter Gorer, and an American geneticist, George Snell, discovered that there were antigens on the surface of red blood cells taken from mice that determined whether or not a graft from one animal would be accepted by another. In 1958, Dausset extended Gorer and Snell's work from mice to men, showing that there were similar antigens on the surface of human tissue cells.
5. In 1969, when only the A and B loci had been discovered, this was known as a '4 antigen' match. With the subsequent discovery of the DR locus, a perfect match became known as a '6 antigen' match.
6. In 1970 the pool of waiting recipients and available kidney donors was so small that a perfectly matched kidney was hardly ever found. Today, with much larger numbers of people, about 10 per cent of kidneys transplanted from unrelated donors (cadavers) will be perfect matches. With kidneys transplanted between very close family members, siblings for example, the figure can rise to 25 per cent. Statistics from UCLA Tissue Typing Laboratory.

7. This is a controversial area. Others who questioned the predictive ability of tissue typing in this period made a distinction between kidneys taken from unrelated cadavers and those transplanted between close blood relatives. They believed tissue matching worked if the donor and recipient were close family members but agreed with Najarian that, in all other circumstances, only a perfect match would significantly increase survival time.

8. Tom Starzl, *The Puzzle People*, p. 122.

9. Ibid., p. 123.

10. He began the work at Stanford University Medical Centre but moved across to the neighbouring Veterans' Administration Hospital where he continued the project in 1969.

11. The skin is the barrier between the body and the outside world. It is designed to keep out bacteria, viruses and other foreign matter. It is perhaps not surprising, therefore, that it provokes a strong immune response when transplanted.

12. Quoted in Joseph Hixson's *The Patchwork Mouse*, pp. 103–4.

13. Ibid., p. 32.

14. Quoted in Joseph Hixson's *The Patchwork Mouse*, p. 41.

15. Ibid., p. 105–6.

16. Ibid., p. 47.

17. Ibid., p. 10.

18. Report of the Summerlin Peer Review Committee, 17 May 1974.

19. While working at the Memorial Hospital, Summerlin transplanted cultured skin onto five patients in an attempt to heal chronic ulcers. In their conclusions the investigating committee noted that 'in four of these five patients there appeared to be an increase in the time during which the graft persisted'. Two of the grafts were still surviving when the committee wrote its report and 'the possibility of a permanent take cannot be ruled out', the report stated.

20. A handful of researchers continued working in the field. One of them, Dr Kevin Lafferty of the Australian National University of Canberra, says that he has since used tissue culturing successfully to prevent rejection in some endocrine organs. William Summerlin was on the right track, says Lafferty, but his technique was wrong. 'Bill Summerlin would never tell me how he was doing his culturing,' he explains. 'So when I was first trying to reproduce his

work, I wrote back to Bill and said, "I cannot do this." He said, "I am sending you a recipe book to tell you how to do it." Of course, the book never turned up . . . so I went to the library and looked up how you culture the thyroid. I thought that thyroid would be very easy to do. The library book says you must culture it in 95 per cent oxygen. Bill and the others were not doing it this way. So I did it because the library book told me to. And it worked.' Lafferty says he can now transplant endocrine organs like the thyroid, pancreatic islets and pituitary gland that can be cut up, cultured and then transplanted. He says that some mice transplanted in this way have survived for two years with no rejection and without the need for any drugs. 'If it was not for him [Summerlin] I would not even have thought of culturing the tissue in this way.'

21. See Chapter 2, pp. 45–46.
22. The British team found a novel way of getting the drug absorbed into the body. They didn't go for chemicals with long names – instead they made use of a gift sent to Alkis Kostakis, a Greek surgeon temporarily in London working with David White. 'His mother thought he might starve to death in England, because the food was so bad here,' explains Sir Roy Calne. 'So she sent him a big can of pure Greek olive oil – and he found this was a marvellous solvent for the drug.'
23. See the paper by R.Y. Calne and D. White in *IRCS Med. Sci.*, 1977, p. 595.
24. See the paper 'Prolonged Survival of Serologically Mismatched Orthotopic Pig Heart Transplants' by R.Y. Calne, D. White *et al.*, published in the *Lancet*, 3 June 1978, pp. 1183–1185.
25. Quoted in 'The Discovery and Development of Cyclosporin' by Jean Borel and Z.L. Kis, in *Transplantation Proceedings*, April 1991, vol. 23, p. 1872. The first clinical use of Cyclosporin was not completely trouble-free, as Calne made clear in a report of these trials published in the *Lancet* in 1979. He had noticed that none of the patients' kidneys worked normally and some even developed a cancer called a lymphoma. But the problem was the amount of drug he was administering. He had given them the same dose as he had his experimental dogs, and this proved much too high. At this level in humans, Cyclosporin has disconcerting side-effects not apparent

in dogs; it damages the kidney; it can cause cancer and excessive hair growth. Once the dosage was reduced, Calne found that Cyclosporin could hold rejection at bay without unduly damaging the body.

26. Statistics from Professor Ferdinand Mühlbacher, University of Vienna. Today the figure has climbed to over 90 per cent.

6. Dying for an Organ

1. Figures taken from the International Transplantation Bulletin Service, August 1994.

2. In 1993, Austria (which has presumed consent) managed to provide 81 per cent more organ donors per million inhabitants than Britain (which does not). Belgium provided nearly 50 per cent more and Finland 30 per cent more than the UK. Figures from the International Transplant Bulletin Service.

3. Although doctors in Spain continue to consult relatives before taking organs from brain-dead patients, this country still manages to provide nearly 50 per cent more donors than countries, like Britain, that also adhere to the 'informed consent' system. The reasons for this success are thought to be connected to the appointment of local transplant co-ordinators and to the relatively high number of fatal road traffic accidents in Spain.

4. France Transplant no longer exists. In 1994 it was replaced by a new national co-ordinating body called L'Etablissement Français des Greffes.

5. *L'Express*, 28 May 1992, p. 74.

6. Ibid., p. 76. It is ironic that, had Christophe died just a few months later, there would have been no need to remove his eyes because a new procedure was introduced, enabling surgeons to remove the corneas without also removing the eyeball. They can then be replaced with a small implant which restores the appearance of the dead person. Amiens Hospital's transplant department began using the new method in January 1992, five months after Christophe's death.

7. The controversy surrounding the Tesniere case was just one of a number of issues that led to the introduction of a new law, which

covers a wide range of issues. Other influential factors were a scandal about organs being sold to hospitals in France, and another row about the transmission of the HIV virus, which resulted in the instigation of criminal proceedings against several government ministers.

8. The law also makes brain-death a legal concept for the first time in India.

9. Todd Leventhal gave an address to the 7th European Congress of the European Society for Organ Transplantation. One sign of just how effective is his anti-organ theft campaign was the press release of his speech. The headline on the two-page summary read: Child Organ Trafficking Exposed as Urban Myth. Without inverted commas around the phrase 'urban myth', one man's opinion had become everyone's fact.

7. A Pig to Save Your Bacon

1. These operations were done by Matthieu Jaboulay and Ernest Unger. See Chapter 1 pages 19 and 20 for a fuller account.

2. From 'The Future of Xenotransplantation' published in *Annals of Surgery*, October 1992, vol. 216, no. 4.

3. Quoted in 'History of Transplantation: 35 Recollections', ed. Paul Terasaki, p. 555.

4. *Time* magazine, 27 December 1963, p. 41.

5. The operations were done with Dr Brian H. McCracken and Dr Jorgen Schlegel.

6. Reemtsma, McCracken *et al.*, 'Renal Heterotransplantation in Man', in *Annals of Surgery*, July–December 1964, vol. 60, p. 405.

7. Hitchcock then joined Tom Starzl's transplant team in Denver, Colorado, and went on to give baboon kidneys to six other patients. They were not hyperacutely rejected but very high doses of drugs were needed to keep the organs functioning. They were eventually rejected within six weeks of the operations. Starzl concluded from this experience that the use of baboon organs would have to wait for better and possibly different immuno-suppression. 'The death of six patients was a devastating loss,' he says. 'We never tried again.' See

'Baboon Renal and Chimpanzee Liver Heterotransplantation' in *Xenograft 25*, ed. Mark A. Hardy, 1989.

8. Letter to Allie Rush, Boyd Rush's second wife, February 1964.

9. Boyd Rush's sister signed a consent form that stated: '. . . If for any unanticipated reason the heart should fail completely during either operation and it should prove impossible to start it, I agree to the insertion of a suitable heart transplant if such should be available at the time. I further understand that hundreds of heart transplants have been performed in laboratories throughout the world but that any heart transplant would represent the initial transplant in man.'

10. According to Hardy, Kolff later asked him if he had realized this. Hardy said, 'No, and I don't think that the world-wide audience knew that you were joking.'

11. James Hardy, *The World of Surgery, 1945–1985. Memoirs of One Participant*, p. 278.

12. Ibid., p. 280.

13. There was a handful of attempts after 1964. Tom Starzl transplanted a chimpanzee's liver into a person on three occasions: in 1966, 1969 and 1973. None of his patients, all young children, lived longer than fourteen days. The Italian surgeon Raffaello Cortesini transplanted one kidney taken from a chimp into a nineteen-year-old man. He died thirty days later, although the chimp lived for a further two years on its remaining kidney. Cortesini did a number of other chimp transplants in the late 1960s and even dallied with the idea of breeding chimpanzees for their organs. Moral disapproval put an end to this idea. In 1977 Christiaan Barnard made two unsuccessful attempts to transplant chimpanzee hearts into humans in South Africa. His first patient, a twenty-six-year-old woman, survived for just six hours. His second, a fifty-nine-year-old man, lived for four days. These were 'piggyback' operations in which the donor's sick heart was left to beat alongside the transplanted heart. Barnard abandoned the technique after these poor results. He also decided not to transplant any more organs from chimpanzees.

14. Loma Linda University was founded in 1906 as the College of Medical Evangelists. It specializes in training Seventh Day Adventists as medical missionaries.

15. Bailey and his colleagues in the department of surgery agreed to

contribute 10 per cent of their incomes towards the animal research to cover an expenditure that ranged from $250,000 to $500,000 each year. There were also a few private cash gifts and donations of equipment, but they covered only a small fraction of the running costs.

16. Its correct title is the Institutional Review Board.

17. *International Herald Tribune*, 29 October 1984.

18. *Guardian*, 29 October 1984.

19. *New York Times*, 6 November 1984.

20. *Time* magazine, 12 November 1984. Najarian either didn't know about Keith Reemtsma's nine-month chimpanzee-kidney survivor, or was dismissing it as a failure.

21. Interviewed on WETA's *MacNeil Lehrer News Hour*, 16 November 1984.

22. The procedure is called the Norwood operation after its inventor Dr William Norwood, of the Children's Hospital in Philadelphia. It involves the construction of an extra pumping chamber on the right side of the heart and the re-routing of the heart's blood supply. In 1984 this was an exceptionally difficult operation with a high mortality rate. Norwood had treated 100 infants in this way of whom only forty had survived. '[The operation] is not a trivial business,' he said at the time, 'and if one intends to have a serious impact on this disease, numerous alternatives have to be explored.'

23. Two years after the Baby Fae operation the Animal Liberation Front broke into the laboratories at the medical centre, released animals and stole research files. The ALF says the documents prove that Bailey's cross-species transplants were not as successful as he has claimed and that he was not ready to try the technique out in a baby.

24. Margo Tannenbaum says she was arrested and charged with receiving property stolen from the medical centre's laboratories. She pleaded not guilty but the charge was dropped on the morning the trial was due to begin.

25. Leonard Bailey has since gone on to pioneer human heart transplants in very young babies. In the past ten years 300 such operations have been done at Loma Linda University. His longest surviving patient was given a new heart in November 1985 at the age of just four days and is now (1995) ten years old.

26. There have been a few unsuccessful attempts to transplant organs from other animals. Although it was known that transplantation of organs across the species barrier consistently failed, Denton Cooley, the cardiac surgeon from Houston in Texas, tried a sheep's heart in 1968 to save a dying man for whom no suitable human donor could be found. The patient died on the operating table. In 1992 Leonard Makowka, in charge of the transplant team at the Cedar-Sinai Medical Centre in Los Angeles, used a pig's liver as a temporary transplant to try to keep a twenty-six-year-old dying woman alive long enough for a suitable human liver to be found. He failed. The woman died thirty hours after the animal's liver was joined in tandem with her own damaged liver after her brain was fatally damaged by a rise in the pressure inside her skull. This is a common complication of liver disease and is caused by unfiltered toxins flowing through the bloodstream into the brain. It is also a sign that the pig's liver was not working properly. Makowka faced considerable flak for his efforts. 'There's absolutely no basis in basic research for trying a pig liver in a human being given the differences in biology between people and pigs,' complained Arthur Caplan, director of the Biomedical Ethics Centre at the University of Minnesota. Makowka was unperturbed by the critics. 'We were faced with a young woman deteriorating before our eyes,' he said, adding that he would do it again in similar circumstances.

27. Imutran began to receive financial backing from the pharmaceutical giant Sandoz nine years after the project had begun.

28. In the centre of every cell in the pigs' bodies are 23 pairs of chromosomes which contain DNA (deoxyribonucleic acid), the genetic code that determines all of an animal's bodily characteristics.

29. It is a difficult procedure. The gene responsible for the protein 'flags' is successfully included in the pig's genetic code only about once in every fifty attempts. Then the egg has to be implanted into the uterus of a sow, a surrogate mother; at this stage, many pregnancies fail.

30. White began using the gene that provides MCP in the pigs in 1994. He has not yet (December 1995) used CD 59.

31. The American firm is taking a slightly different technical approach

to the problem of hyperacute rejection from its English competitor. Alexion Pharmaceuticals are engineering their pigs with a complement-inhibitor that they've made themselves and which combines the functions of DAF and CD 59. They are also engineering the animals with a human blood-group enzyme that they think will also help to prevent hyperacute rejection. The Americans believe this dual approach will be more effective than that being taken by Imutran. So far (December 1995) they have only introduced their complement-inhibitor into the animals.

8. Brave New Bodies

1. Quoted in *The Plain Dealer*, 10 May 1988.
2. Quoted in *The American Scholar*, 1971, vol. 40, no. 3.
3. He used rhesus monkeys. He also used dogs in these early experiments but it quickly became apparent that it was much easier anatomically and surgically to isolate the monkey brain.
4. In an article published in 1982 White gives a more detailed description of the state of awareness of his transplanted monkey head: he calls it a 'cephalon'. 'In the ensuing hours following surgery, a completely awake state supervened . . . It was obvious the animals could see and did appreciate movement . . . if a loud sound was produced, the cephalon evidenced by a facial expression of discomfort. Light pinprick on the facial tissues, likewise, gave evidence of discomfort on the part of the animal. These preparations could and did masticate and swallow food as well as appropriately handling fluids employing the expected muscle movements of tongue and oral cavity. Indeed one had the impression that the animals were "hungry and thirsty" and understood the oral processing of food and liquid with alacrity.' See R.J. White, 'Experimental Transference of Consciousness: the Human Equivalent' in J. Eccles (ed.), *Mind and Brain: the Many-faceted Problems* pp.147–50.
5. In later whole body transplants, the heads were able to breathe unaided. In these experiments (he calls them his more advanced model), White preserved the brain stem – the part of the brain responsible for respiration – and transplanted it with the body.

6. Hans Ruesch, *The Naked Empress: All the Great Medical Fraud*, Civis, Zurich, 1982.
7. 3 September 1993.
8. 6 September 1993.
9. *Independent on Sunday*, 5 September 1993.
10. *Daily Telegraph*, 13 September 1993.
11. *Daily Telegraph*, 13 November 1993.
12. The protein alpha-antitrypsin is a substance made in the liver that plays an important role in preventing the breakdown of enzymes in various organs of the body. If the level of alpha-antitrypsin falls too low it can damage the liver, scarring it and making it function abnormally.
13. A study on 529 liver transplant patients conducted by the US Multicentre FK506 Liver Study Group at Baylor University Medical Centre in Dallas showed that 82 per cent of livers transplanted into patients given FK506 survived for one year compared to 79 per cent of livers in patients given Cyclosporin. Information from *International Transplantation Bulletin*, September 1994.
14. The Broward edition of the *Miami Herald*, 21 August 1994.
15. Associated Press report, 13 June 1994.
16. Quoted in the Broward edition of the *Miami Herald*, 21 August 1994.
17. Ibid.
18. Since Benito's death, Pittsburgh Children's Hospital have introduced a number of methods to try to ensure that there is no repeat of the Agrelo incident. They say they are now much more attentive to the complaints of their young patients – putting them on a different medicine if the side-effects are too severe and reducing the dosage of anti-rejection drugs as far as possible. They have also established a four-day holiday camp where seven- to seventeen-year-old transplant patients can get to know one another. 'We hope that friendships will begin at the camp so that these patients will have someone to turn to in a crisis – and that person will also be a transplant patient,' explains Jorge Reyes.

Postscript: The Mystery of Betty's Body

1. R.Y. Calne, H.J.O. White, D.E. Yoffa *et al.*, 'Prolonged Survival of Liver Transplants in the Pig', *British Medical Journal*, 16 December 1967, p. 648. This paper reported on a series of thirty-six liver transplants in pigs. Calne had already done nineteen other liver transplants in pigs with similar results. The conclusions in this earlier series of experiments were published in the *BMJ* on 20 May 1967, pp. 478–480. He later wrote a third paper stating overall conclusions about the two series of experimental transplants. This was published in *Transplantation Proceedings*, March 1969, vol. 1, no. 1, pp. 321–4.
2. The experiment is described more fully in Chapter 2 on pp. 38–41.
3. See pages 106–07.
4. According to Tom Starzl, five of the world's ten longest-surviving transplant patients have not taken immuno-suppressant drugs for considerable periods of time. He also thinks that some people given other organs have come off their drugs as well, but that such cases have yet to be properly documented.
5. These two processes are respectively called 'Host versus Graft (HVG)' and 'Graft versus Host (GVH)' reactions. See T.E. Starzl *et al.*, 'Cell Migration, Chimerism and Graft Acceptance', *The Lancet*, 339: 1579–82, 1992.

Bibliography

BOOKS

Barnard, C. and Pepper, C.B., *One Life*, George C. Harrap & Co., London, 1970

Barnard, C., *The Second Life*, Vlaeberg Publishers, Cape Town, 1993

Blaiberg, P., *Looking at my Heart*, William Heinemann Ltd, London, 1969

Hamilton, D., *The Monkey Gland Affair*, Chatto & Windus, London, 1986

Hardy, J., *The World of Surgery, 1945–1985. Memoirs of One Participant*, University of Pennsylvania Press, Philadelphia, 1986

Hixson, J., *The Patchwork Mouse*, Anchor Press and Doubleday, New York, 1970

Kuss, R. and Bourget, P., *An Illustrated History of Organ Transplantation*, Sandoz, Rueil-Malmaison, France, 1992

Malinin, T., *Surgery and Life – The Extraordinary Career of Alexis Carrel*, Harcourt Brace Jovanovich, New York and London, 1979

Medawar, Sir P., *Memoir of a Thinking Radish*, Oxford University Press, Oxford, 1988

Moore, F.D., *A Miracle and a Privilege: Recounting a Half Century of Surgical Advance*, Joseph Henry Press, Washington DC, 1995

Moore, F.D., *Transplant: the Give and Take of Tissue Transplantation*, Simon & Schuster, New York, 1972

Neuhof, H., *Transplantation of Tissues*, Appleton & Co., New York, 1923

Starzl, T.E., *Experience in Renal Transplantation*, WB Saunders Company, Philadelphia, London and Toronto, 1964

Starzl, T.E., *The Puzzle People: Memoirs of a Transplant Surgeon*, University of Pittsburgh Press, Pittsburgh, 1993

Terasaki, P. (ed.), *History of Transplantation: 35 Recollections*, UCLA Tissue Typing Laboratory, Los Angeles, 1991

Stirling Edwards, W. and Edwards, P.D., *Alexis Carrel – Visionary Surgeon*, Charles C. Thomas, Illinois, 1974

Thompson, T., *Hearts – Debakey & Cooley, Surgeons Extraordinary*, Michael Joseph, London, 1972

PAPERS

Billingham, R.E., Brent, L. and Medawar, P., 'Actively Acquired Tolerance of Foreign Cells', *Nature*, 1953, vol. 172, pp. 603–06

Borel, J.F. and Kis, Z.L., 'The Discovery and Development of Cyclosporin', *Transplantation Proceedings*, April 1991, vol. 23, no. 2, pp. 1867–1874

Calne, R.Y., 'The Rejection of Renal Homografts. Inhibition in Dogs by 6-Mercaptopurine', *Lancet*, 20 February 1960, pp. 417–418

Calne, R.Y., 'Inhibition of the Rejection of Renal Homografts by Purine Analogues', *Transplantation Bulletin*, October 1961, vol. 28, no. 2

Calne, R.Y., White, H.J.O. *et al.*, 'Observations of Orthotopic Liver Transplantation in the Pig', *British Medical Journal*, 20 May 1967, vol. 2, pp. 478–480

Calne, R.Y., White, H.J.O. *et al.*, 'Prolonged Survival of Liver Transplants in the Pig', *British Medical Journal*, 16 December 1967, vol. 4, pp. 645–648

Calne, R.Y., White, H.J.O. *et al.*, 'Immunosuppressive Effects of the Orthotopically Transplanted Porcine Liver', *Transplantation Proceedings*, March 1969, vol. 1, no. 1, pp. 321–324

Calne, R.Y., White, D.J.G. *et al.*, 'Cyclosporin A – A Powerful Immunosuppressant in Dogs with Renal Allografts', IRCS Med. Sci., 1977, 5:595

Calne, R.Y., White, D. and Thiru *et al.*, 'Prolonged Survival of Serologically Mismatched Orthotopic Pig Heart Transplants', *Lancet*, 3 June 1978, pp. 1183–1185

Carrel, A., 'Transplantation in Mass of the Kidneys', *Journal of Experimental Medicine*, 1908

Gibson, T., Medawar, P., 'The Fate of Skin Homografts in Man', *Journal of Anatomy*, London 1943

Hamburger, J., Vaysse, J. *et al.*, 'Renal Transplantation in Man After

Radiation of the Recipient', *American Journal of Medicine*, June 1962, vol. 32, pp. 854–871

Hopewell, J., Calne, R.Y. and Beswick, I., 'Three Clinical Cases of Renal Transplantation', *British Medical Journal*, 15 February 1964, vol. I, pp. 411–413

Hume, D.M., Merrill, J.P., Miller, B.J. and Thorn, G.W., 'Experiences with Renal Homotransplantation in the Human: Report of Nine Cases', *Journal of Clinical Investigation*, February 1955, vol. 34, pp. 327–382

Jaboulay, M., 'Kidney Grafts in the antecubital fossa by arterial and venous anastomosis', *Lyon Medical*, 1906, 107:575

Kuss, R., Teinturier, J. and Millez, P., 'Some Experiments on Renal Grafting In Man', *Mémoires de L'Academie de Chirurgie*, 1951, 77:755

Kuss, R., Legrain, M.D. *et al.*, 'Homologous Human Kidney Transplantation. Experience with six patients', *Postgraduate Medical Journal*, 1962, vol. 38, pp. 528–536

Lawler, R.H., West, J.W. *et al.*, 'Homotransplantation of the Kidney in the Human – A Preliminary Report', *Journal of the American Medical Association*, 4 November 1950, vol. 144, pp. 344 and 345

Lawler, R.H., West, J.W. *et al.*, 'Homotransplantation of the Kidney in the Human – Supplemental Report of a Case', *Journal of the American Medical Association*, 1 September 1951, vol. 147, pp. 45 and 46

Murray, J.E., Merrill, J.P. *et al.*, 'Kidney Transplantation Between Seven Pairs of Identical Twins', *Annals of Surgery*, July–December 1958, vol. 148, pp. 343–356

Murray, J.E., Merrill, J.P. *et al.*, 'Kidney Transplantation in Modified Recipients', *Annals of Surgery*, September 1962, 156:337, pp. 337–355

Merrill, J.P., Murray, J.E. *et al.*, 'Successful Transplantation of Kidney from Human Cadaver', *Journal of the American Medical Association*, 3 August 1963, vol. 185, pp. 347–353

Merrill, J.P., Murray, J.E. *et al.*, 'Successful Homotransplantation of the Human Kidney Between Identical Twins', *Journal of the American Medical Association*, 28 January 1956, pp. 374–379

Murray, J., Wilson, R.E. *et al.*, 'Five Years' Experience with Renal Transplantation with Immunosuppressive Drugs', *Annals of Surgery*, July–December 1968, vol. 168, pp. 416–433

Reemtsma, K., McCracken, B.H. *et al.*, 'Renal Heterotransplantation in Man', *Annals of Surgery*, July–December 1964, vol. 160, pp. 384–410

Schwartz, R. and Damashek, W., 'Drug Induced Immunologic Tolerance', *Nature*, June 1959, vol. 183, p. 1682

Starzl, T.E., Marchioro, T.L., Waddell, W.R., 'The Reversal of Rejection in Human Renal Homografts with Subsequent Development of Homograft Tolerance', *Surgery, Gynaecology and Obstetrics*, October 1963, vol. 117, pp. 385–395

Starzl, T.E., 'The Future of Xenotransplantation', *Annals of Surgery*, October 1992, vol. 216, no. 4

Unger, E., 'Kidney Transplantation', *Klin*, Wochenschr., 1910, translated from German by Ronald G. Landes

Voronoy, Y.Y., 'Blocking the reticulo-endothelial system in man in some forms of mercuric chloride intoxication and the transplantation of the cadaver kidney as a method of treatment for the aneuria resulting from the intoxication', *Siglo Medico*, 1937, 97:296

White, R., 'Experimental Transference of Consciousness: The Human Equivalent' in J. Eccles (ed.) *Mind and Brain: The Many-faceted Problems*, Paragon House, Washington DC, 1982, pp. 147–50

Index

ALG *see* antilymphocyte globulin
Academy of Medicine, Cleveland, Ohio, 181
Actinomycin C, 48n
Addenbrooke's Hospital, Cambridge, 2, 212
Agrelo, Benito,
— hereditary liver disease, 195
— family, 196–9, 201–3
— liver transplants
  first two, 195–6
  drug therapy, 195–7
  refusal of: drugs, 198; third transplant, 200–201
— court hearing, 201
— death, 202–3
Ahmed, Dr Syed Adil, 148
Alexion (American pharmaceutical company), 176 *and* n; 177, 178
Alexis Carrel – Visionary Surgeon (Thomas), 10n
alpha-antitrypsin deficiency (liver defect at birth), 195
American
— Cancer Society, 117
— College of Cardiology, 104
— Information Agency, 153
— Society for Clinical Investigation, 120
— Urological Association, 28
anastomosis (sewing together blood vessels), 3, 8–10, 13
anencephalitis (brain defect at birth), 73

animal rights activists, 12, 154, 166, 167, 172, 185
animals,
— experiments on
  baboons, 158 *and* n; 162, 164–9
  cattle, skin of, 39–40
  chimpanzees, 156–61, 162n
  dogs, 10, 11, 46, 58, 70, 72, 130
  goats, 155
  mice, skin of, 40
  monkeys, 156, 182–4
  pigs, 19–21, 130, 155, 176–7
— transplants from
  disease problems, 174
  moral/ethical problems, 168–9
Annals of Surgery, 156n, 158n
antilymphocyte globulin (ALG), 54, 102n
anti-vivisectionists, 12
Argentina, 152
artificial kidney machines, 2, 31 *and* n; 42, 89, 193–4
Austria, 137 *and* n
azathioprine (Imuran), 46, 54

BSE *see* bovine spongiform encephalopathy
baboons, experiments as organ donors, 158 *and* n; 163, 164–9
'Baby Fae', 164–9
Bailey, Leonard, 163–9, 169n, 179
Baird, Betty, 106–7, 205–6
Bangalore (India), 152
Barnard, Professor Christiaan,
— animal experiments, 58

— celebrity, 67, 83–5
— divorce, 87
— heart transplants
    first, 1, 57–68, 79–83
    further experience, 101–3
— honours, 85
— kidney transplant, 58
— 'Man with the Golden Hands', 60
— perfectionist, 57
Barnard, Karen, 87
Barnard, Louwtjie, 84, 85, 87
Barnes, Dr John
Baylor University, Dallas, 196n
Belgium, 137 *and* n
Bell, Leonard, 178
Beth Israel Hospital, Newark, 166
biliary atresia (liver defect at birth), 53
Billingham, Rupert, 40
Bioethics Law (France), 142
Biomedical Ethics Centre, University of
    Minnesota, 170n
Birkin, Judge Arthur, 201
Blaiberg, Dr Philip, 101–3, 102n
blood vessels, 8–10, 13
Borel, Jean, 128, 129–31
bovine spongiform encephalopathy
    (BSE), 174
bowel defects, 57, 190
Bradley, Bill, 69–70
brain,
— defects at birth, 73
— experiments on monkeys, 182–4
brain-death, 62, 71–2, 88, 137, 138,
    145n
Brent, Leslie, 40, 53, 118–19
Brigham and Women's Hospital,
    Boston, 29n
Bright's disease (glomerulonephritis), 2,
    31 *and* n; 34, 49
Brinkley, John R, 14, 19
British
— Medical Journal, 46n, 204 *and* n
— Society of Immunology, 128

Broussais Hospital, Paris, 29
Brown-Séquard, Charles Edouard, 14
Buffalo Evening News, 118

Caillavet Law (France), 140, 141, 142
California Organ Replacement Agency,
    167
Calne, Sir Roy, 2–3, 40, 45, 46, 48,
    128–30, 191, 204, 207–8
Cambridge University, 107
Cape Times, 67
Caplan, Arthur, 170n
Carnot, President Sadi, 7, 8, 22
Carrel, Alexis,
— lecturer at Lyon University, 9–10
— Nobel Prize in Medicine, 11, 13
— surgeon in Lyon, 7–8
— technique of sewing together blood
    vessels, 9–10
— threats by animal rights activists, 12
— transplants of animal kidneys, 10–11
Caserio, Santo, 7
Case Western Reserve University, Ohio,
    181
Casey, Sister J., 26
Catholic Church, 142, 185
cattle, experiments on, 39–40
Cedar-Sinai Medical Centre, Los
    Angeles, 170n
Central Red Cross Hospital, Spain, 67
'cephalon' (animal's head), 182–3, 184n
Chase, Merrill, 11
Chicago University, 25, 211
Children's Hospital, Cincinnati, 210
chimpanzees, experiments as organ
    donors, 156–61, 162n
Civitas (anti-vivisection movement),
    184
Cochin Hospital, Paris, 29
Colorado University, 126n, 210, 211
complement (toxic protein in the
    blood), 171
Compton, Justice A. Christian, 98–100

Cooley, Denton, 92, 94–5, 170n
Cornell-New York Hospital, 120, 121
cortisone, 106
cross-species transplants, 156, 158, 163,
    166, 168, 176–7, 204–5
Cushing's syndrome (drug side-effect),
    107
Cyclosporin A,
— anti-flammatory agent, 130
— anti-rejection drug, 129–30
— side effects, 133
— use on transplant patients, 131–4,
    168, 196, 208
cystic fibrosis (lung disease), 5, 135

DNX (American biotechnology
    company), 178
Dalton, Fred, 43
Dalton, Roy, 42–3
Darvall, Denise, 55–7, 61–6, 69
Darvall, Edward, 62–3
Dausset, Jean, 108
Davies, Laura, 190–94
Davies, Les and Frances, 190–94
Davis, Jefferson, 156–7
death, definition of,
— 'brain-death', 62, 71–2, 88, 99, 137,
    138, 145n
— in law, 96, 99
— 'point of death', 61
— when heart stops, 64, 71–2
Declerk, Sister Georgie, 56, 79
Dhonpal, Dr Dilip, 147, 148
diabetes, 5
dialysis, 31, 31n, 42, 89, 193–4
*The Discovery and Development of
    Cyclosporin* (Borel and Kis),
    131n
disease problems in transplants from
    animals, 174
Dobson, Sergeant Roy, 199
dogs, experiments on, 10–11, 46, 58,
    70, 72, 130

donor cards, 137
donors of organs *see* organ donors
drug therapy,
— cortisone, 106–7
— Cyclosporin A, 129–34, 168, 195,
    208
— FK506, 191, 193, 196 *and* n
— Imuran, 46, 54, 107, 130
— side effects, 50, 106–7
— 6–MP, 45 *and* n; 46 *and* n; 47, 49,
    50
— *see also* immunology
D'Souza, Inspector Vincent, 148–9
Dubost, Charles, 29, 30
Dubyagin, Colonel Yuri Petrovich, 152

Eames, Malcolm, 155, 173, 174
Ebstein's anomaly, 57
Encyclopaedia Britannica, 18
English, Sir Terence, 92n
Essen University, Germany, 214
European Society for Organ
    Transplantation, 153
Eurotransplant, 137
experiments on,
— baboons, 158 *and* n; 163, 164–9
— cattle, 39–40
— chimpanzees, 156–61, 162n
— dogs, 10–11, 46, 58, 70, 72, 130
— goats, 155
— mice, 40
— monkeys, 156, 182–4
— pigs, 19–21, 130, 155, 176–7
eyes, transplants of, 138–41, 141n, 152

FK506, anti-rejection drug, 191, 193,
    196 *and* n
Face the Nation (TV programme), 84
Fadali, Dr Moneim, 179, 203
Fahd, King of Saudi Arabia, 191
Finland, 138 *and* n
Fisher, Dorothy, 103
Foch Hospital, Paris, 210

Fodor, William, 177
Forde, Gordon, 91
France: transplant legalities, 138,
    140–42
France Transplant, 139 *and* n
Friedmann, Dene, 57, 66, 67, 80
The Future of Xenotransplantation
    (Starzl), 156n

gastroschisis (bowel defect at birth),
    190
genetic engineering, 155, 170–71,
    172–3, 174–7
Genetics Forum, 155, 173
Germany, 137
Gibson, Tom, 23
gland grafting,
— 'Glandular' fever, 16
— monkey glands, 16–17
— testis gland, 13–15
Glasgow Royal Infirmary, 23
glomerulonephritis (Bright's disease), 2,
    31 *and* n; 34, 49
goats, experiments on, 155
Good, Professor Robert, 116–19,
    120–21, 122–3, 125
Gordon, Anne, 101, 103
Gould, Dr Donald, 91
Great Karoo (South Africa), 84n
Groote Schuur Hospital, Cape Town,
    56–8, 66, 67, 77, 79, 80, 102
Grundon, Ron, 133
Guardian, 165n
Guillot, Dolly, 92
Guy's Hospital, London, 2, 45

HLA *see* human leukocyte antigen
Hague, The (Holland), 111
Haller, Jordan, 75–6
Hamburger, Professor Jean, 29, 30, 35,
    42, 49–50, 51, 52
Hamilton, David, 16, 18
Hamilton, Sherry, 180

Hardy, James, 158–62
Harefield Hospital, Uxbridge, 92n
Haupt, Clive, 102
Health and Rehabilitative Services
    (Florida), 199–200
Heart Centre, North Rhine Westphalia,
    Germany, 210
heart-lung,
— machines, 65, 160
— transplants, 132–3
hearts, transplants of,
— from anencephalitic infants, 73–8
— to babies, 164–9, 169n
— from baboons, 164–9
— from chimpanzees, 156–8
— early failures, 88–91
— emotional reactions to, 69
— first, 57–68, 79–83
— further experiences, 101–4
— in Japan, 100–101
— legal problems, 98–9, 100
— survival rates, 104
— survival records, 210
Hendrick, Charles, 91
Herrick, Richard, 34–8
Herrick, Ronald, 34–8
*History of Transplantation: 35
    Recollections* (Terasaki), 50n
Hitchcock, Claude, 158
'Holy Grail' of transplantation, 208
hospitals,
— Addenbrooke's Hospital,
    Cambridge, 2, 212
— Beth Israel Hospital, Newark, 166
— Brigham and Women's Hospital,
    Boston, 29n
— Broussais Hospital, Paris, 29
— Cedar-Sinai Medical Centre, Los
    Angeles, 170n
— Central Red Cross Hospital, Spain,
    68
— Children's Hospital, Cincinnati, 210
— Cochin Hospital, Paris, 29

— Cornell-New York Hospital, 120, 121
— Foch Hospital, Paris, 210
— Glasgow Royal Infirmary, 23
— Groote Schuur Hospital, Cape Town, 56–8, 66, 67, 77, 79, 80, 102
— Guy's Hospital, London, 2, 45
— Harefield Hospital, Uxbridge, 92n
— Heart Centre, North Rhine Westphalia, Germany, 210
— Jackson Memorial Hospital, Miami, 195, 200
— Lady Willingdon Hospital, Madras, 143
— Little Company of Mary Hospital, Chicago, 26, 28
— Madras Government Hospital, 145
— Maimonides Medical Centre, New York, 72, 74
— Massachusetts General Hospital, 10, 119
— Mayo Clinic, Minnesota, 213
— Medical College of Virginia, 58, 96–7
— Memorial Sloan-Kettering Cancer Centre Hospital, New York, 116
— National Heart Hospital, London, 68, 69
— Necker Hospital, Paris, 29, 30, 49, 52, 210, 212
— North Indiana Heart Institute, 211
— Papworth Hospital, Cambridge, 92n, 136, 170
— Peter Bent Brigham Hospital, Boston, 29, 31, 34–8, 42, 46
— Pittsburgh Children's Hospital, 191, 195
— Radcliffe Infirmary, Oxford, 22
— Red Cross Hospital, Lyon, 8
— Royal Free Hospital, London, 45
— St. Luke's Hospital, Houston, 92, 93
— St Mary's Hospital, Manchester, 190
— Sapporo Medical College, Japan, 100
— Stanford University Medical Centre, San Francisco, 70, 104, 114, 115, 133, 211, 213
— Texas Heart Institute, Houston, 210
— Toronto General Hospital, Canada, 211
— University Hospital of North Amiens, France, 138–40
— Veterans' Administration Hospital, Denver, 48, 53, 110
— Victoria Hospital, Bangalore, 147
— Yelamma Desappa Hospital, India, 147, 150
Houssin, Professor Didier, 141–2
human leukocyte antigen (HLA), 108n
Hume, David, 29, 31–3, 58
hydrocephalus, 29
Hyett, Stephen, 2–3, 4
Hygeia (American Medical Association Journal), 19
hyperacute rejection of organs, 20, 156, 170–71
hypoplastic left-heart syndrome (heart defect at birth), 164, 167n

Illustrated History of Organ Transplantation (Küss), 13n, 30n
immunology,
— animal experiments, 39–40, 46, 130, 204–5
— bone marrow replacement, 41–3
— drug therapy
ALG, 53
cortisone, 106
Cyclosporin A, 129–34, 168, 195, 208
FK506, 191, 193, 196 *and* n
Prednisone, 48–9
side effects, 50, 106
6-MP, 45 *and* n; 46 *and* n; 47, 49, 50

— survival of transplants without
drugs, 206–8
— tissue-typing, 107–114
— work by Medawar, 22–4, 39–41, 51,
120
— X-ray radiation, 41–4, 46
— *see also* rejection of organs tissue
typing
Imuran (azathioprine), 46, 54, 106, 107
Imutran (genetic engineering
company), 155, 171, 177
Independent, 192
India,
— sale of organs for transplant
court action, 152
legality of, 145–6
price, 144
— transplant programme, 143
Innsbruck University, Austria, 213
International Herald Tribune, 165n
International Transplantation Bulletin,
136n, 138n, 196n
International Transplantation Society,
154
intestinal atresia (bowel defect), 57
Iwasaki, Dr Yuji, 101n

Jaboulay, Dr Mathieu, 19–20, 156n
Jackson Memorial Hospital, Miami,
195, 200
Japan: transplant surgery and religion,
100–101
Johnson, President Lyndon B., 84
Journal of Experimental Medicine, 11n,
124

Kansas Star (newspaper), 118
Kantrowitz, Adrian, 72–8, 87–8
Kaplan, Barry, 59
Kasperak, Mike, 88
Kettering Laboratory, 122
kidneys,
— artificial, 2, 31 *and* n; 42, 89, 193–4

— transplants of
animal, 10 *and* n; 11, 19–21, 156,
158 *and* n; 159–62
human: initial attempts, 21, 26–8,
30, 31; first success, 31–2;
survival rates, 44, 48, 58;
between twins, 34–8
kidneys, transplants of,
— survival records, 210
Kidney Transplantation (Unger), 20n
Kiev, Ukraine, 189
Kis, Z. L., 131n
Klebsiella (micro-organism), 81
Klett, Joseph, 97, 99n
Kolff, Dr Wilhelm, 162
Küss, René, 29, 30, 31, 42, 44, 47, 52

Lady Willingdon Hospital, Madras, 143
Lafay Law (France), 140, 141
Lafferty, Dr Kevin, 126n
Laino, Dr Peter, 120, 121, 125
Lancet (medical journal), 45n, 204
La Républicain (newspaper), 7
Lawler, Dr Richard H., 25–30
legal problems in transplantation, 98–9,
100, 140–41
Le Monde (newspaper), 51
Le Quotidien du Médicine (medical
journal), 52
L'Etablissement Français des Greffes,
139n, 140, 141
leukaemia, 5
Leventhal, Todd, 153
limbs, amputated, 10
Little Company of Mary Hospital,
Chicago, 26, 28
liver defect at birth, 195
livers, transplants of, 53, 54, 101n,
106–7, 196n, 196–207, 204n,
211
Lollobrigida, Gina, 86–7
Loma Linda University, Los Angeles,
163 *and* n; 164, 165, 210

London University, 40
Longmore, Donald, 68–70, 90
Looking at my Heart (Blaiberg), 102n
Losman, Jacques, 167
Lower, Richard, 96–8, 99n
Lowman, Gladys, 42, 43
Loyola University, Chicago, 25
lung,
— disease, 5, 135
— transplants of, 211
Luxembourg, 137
Lydston, George Frank, 16
Lyon University, 9, 10

Madras Government Hospital, 145
Maimonides Medical Centre, New
    York, 72, 74
Makowka, Leonard, 170n
Malathi (Indian slumdweller), 144
'Man with the Golden Hands', 60
Marcus, Dr Abraham, 91
Martin, James, 122
Massachusetts General Hospital, 10,
    119
Maxwell, Margaret, 192
Mayo Clinic, Minnesota, 213
McCracken, Dr Brian H., 157n
Medawar, Sir Peter,
— Nobel Prize in Medicine (1960), 51
— pioneer in immunology, 24, 39, 41
— skin grafts, 22–3, 40, 120
— 'Trojan Horse' prevention of organ
    rejection, 40–41, 204
Medical College of Virginia, 58, 96–7
medical ethics, 35, 77, 168
Medical Research Council, 23, 171
Medical World News, 25n
Memoir of a Thinking Radish
    (Medawar), 22n, 39n
Memorial Sloan-Kettering Cancer
    Centre Hospital, New York, 117
mice, experiments on, 40
Milford, Kansas, 14–15

Miller, Dr David C., 34
Miller, George, 115, 118, 125
Minnesota University, 108, 116, 212
Mississipi University, 158, 161
Mondino, Dr Bartley, 120, 125
Monkey Gland Affair (Hamilton), 16n,
    18n
monkey glands, 16–17
monkeys, experiments on, 156, 182–4
Moore, Francis, 32, 41–2, 44, 54, 89, 96
moral/ethical problems in
    transplantation, 1, 5, 168–9,
    185–6
Morris, Rustin, 135–6
Muggeridge, Malcolm, 91
Mühlbacher, Professor Ferdinand, 133n
multiple organ transplants, 2–3, 4, 63,
    138, 139–40, 191, 212–14
Murray, Joseph,
— initial work with twins, 33, 35
— suppression of immune system,
    42–4, 46, 47
— Nobel Prize in Medicine (1990), 51,
    52
Mutthusethupathi, Dr M.A., 145

NIH *see* National Institutes of Health
Najarian, Dr John, 108–9, 112, 167
The Naked Empress (Ruesch), 184n
National Heart Hospital, London, 68,
    70
National Institutes of Health (NIH),
    112–13, 121, 122
National Research Council
    (Washington DC), 47
Necker Hospital, Paris, 29, 30, 49, 52,
    210, 212
Nehlsen-Cannarella, Sandra, 165
Netherlands, 137
Neuhof, Harold, 21
New Scientist (magazine), 91
Newsweek magazine, 27
New York Daily News, 67

New York Times, 19, 27, 118, 165n
Ninnemann, John, 119, 120, 121, 123
Nobel Prizes in Medicine, 11, 13 *and* n;
    23, 51, 52, 53, 108
Nobuo, Miyazaki, 100
Nora, Jim, 92, 95
North Indiana Heart Institute, 211
Norwood, Dr William, 167n

Observer, 91, 192
One Life (Barnard and Pepper), 55n
opt-out system for organ donors, 137–8
organ donors,
— donor cards, 137
— eyes, 138–41, 141n, 152
— hearts
  baboons, 163
  chimpanzees, 158–62
  Darvall, Denise, 63–6
  Haupt, Clive, 102
  pigs, 176–7
  Senz, Ralph, 75–6
  Tucker, Bruce, 96–8
— kidneys
  baboons, 158 *and* n
  chimpanzees, 156–8
  French prisoners, 30 *and* n
  identical twins, 34–8
  tissue matching, 33
  Velu (Indian labourer), 147–51
— lack of, 26, 29, 134, 137
— live, 30, 137
— multiple organs, 2–3, 4, 63, 138,
    139–40, 191
— opt-out system, 137–8
Ortiz, Marcelo, 152
Oxford University, 22

pancreas, transplants of, 3, 5, 101n, 211
Papworth Hospital, Cambridge, 92n,
    136, 170
paralysis, 187–8, 189
Parkinson's disease, 5

The Patchwork Mouse (Hixson), 121n
patents in genetic engineering, 177–8
patients,
— heart
  'Baby Fae', 164–9
  Blaiberg, Dr Philip, 101–3
  Fisher, Dorothy, 103
  Forde, Gordon, 91
  Hendrick, Charles, 91
  Kasperak, Mike, 88
  Klett, Joseph, 97
  Nobuo, Miyazaki, 100
  Rush, Boyd, 159–61
  Thomas, Everett, 92
  Van Zyl, Dirk, 103
  Washkansky, Louis, 56–67, 79–83
— heart-lung
  Grundon, Roy, 132–3
— kidney
  Davis, Jefferson, 156–7
  Herrick, Richard, 34–8
  Lowman, Gladys, 42, 43
  Thiebault, Yvette, 49
  Tucker, Ruth, 25–8
  Ustipak, Lorraine, 108–9
— liver
  Agrelo, Benito, 195–203
  Baird, Betty, 106–7, 205–6
— multiple organs
  Davies, Laura, 191
  Hyett, Stephen, 2–3, 4
— whole-body
  Vetovite, Craig, 187–8
— waiting lists of, 5, 136
Patil, Dr Dilip, 147
Peter Bent Brigham Hospital, Boston,
    29, 31, 34–8, 42, 46
Phillips, Melanie, 192
philosophy of transplants, 178–9, 186,
    203
pigs,
— experiments on, 19–21, 130, 155,
    176–7

— liver transplants between, 204n, 204–5
— organs for transplants, 154–5, 170, 172, 175
Pittsburgh Children's Hospital, 191, 195
Pittsburgh University, 54, 206, 211, 212, 213, 214
Prednisone, 49, 54
proteins: complement-blocking, 171, 178
The Puzzle People: Memoirs of a Transplant Surgeon (Starzl), 48n, 113n

quadriplegia (paralysis), 187–8, 189
Queen's Medical Centre, Nottingham, 137

Raaf, John, 119, 121, 123
Radcliffe Infirmary, Oxford, 22
Red Cross Hospital, Lyon, France, 8
Reddy, Dr K.C., 143, 145–6
Reemtsma, Keith, 156–8, 159
rejection of organs,
— between animals and humans, 19–20
— hearts, 94–5
— hyperacute, 19–20, 156, 170–71
— by immune system, 4
— kidneys
   animal, 11–13, 39
   human, 28, 30
— livers, pig, 204–5
— testes, 14
— *see also* drug therapy; immunology
Renal Heterotransplantation in Man (Reemtsma, McCracken), 158n
Renard, Marius, 30, 35
Reyes, Dr Jorge, 196, 199
Riteris, John, 44
Roberts, Catherine, 181
Rockefeller Institute, New York, 11

Rogers, Arkansas, 126
Romano, Dr Phillippe, 140
Rose-Innes, Dr Peter, 61–2
Ross, Donald, 90n
Royal Army Medical Corps, 45
Royal Free Hospital, London, 45
Royal Veterinary College, 69
Ruesch, Hans, 184 *and* n
Rush, Boyd, 159–61
Russia, 152

St Luke's Hospital, Houston, 92, 93
St Mary's Hospital, Manchester, 190
sale of organs for transplant,
— court action, 152
— legality of, 145–6
— price, 144
Sandoz (Swiss pharmaceutical company),
— search for immuno-suppressive compounds, 127
— Cyclosporin A
   production of, 127–8, 131
   side effects from, 133
   use, 131–4, 168, 195
— support for genetic engineeering, 155
San Quentin Prison, California, 15–16
Sant Prison, Paris, 30
Sapporo Medical College, Japan, 100
Saudi Arabia, 191
Schlegel, Dr Jorgan, 157n
Schrire, Professor Velva, 58–9
Scientific American, 18
Scudero, Ann, 77
Scudero, Jamie, 77, 88
The Second Life (Barnard), 57n
Senz, Ralph, 75–6
Senz, Rhoda and Richard, 74–5
Servelle, Marceau, 29, 30
Shumway, Dr Norman, 71–3, 88, 104
Siddaraju, Dr K.S., 147–9, 151
Siméon, Georges, 44

6-mercaptopurine (6–MP), 45 *and* n; 46 *and* n; 47, 49, 50

Sixth International Transplantation Conference, New York, 161–2

skin grafts, 22–4, 40, 114–23

— *see also* tissue typing

Sklar, Grace, 56

Sloan-Kettering Institute, 116–18, 120, 126

Smith, Prentiss, 157

Société de Biologie, Paris, 14

Spain, 138 *and* n

spare-part surgery *see* transplants

Stahelin, Hartmann, 127–8

Stanford University Medical Centre, San Francisco, 70, 104, 114, 115, 133, 211, 213

Stanley, Dr Leo, 15–16, 18

Starzl, Tom,

— transplants

    kidney, 48, 48n, 53

    liver, 53, 110, 112, 206–7

Stevenson, Miller, 74–7

Stinton, Ed, 72

Stritch School of Medicine, Loyola University, 25

Summerlin, Dr William,

— burns, treatment of, 114

— early work, 114–16

— skin grafts, tissues apparently not rejected, 116

— extended experiments, 116–17

— criticism of work, 119–23

— faking of results, 122–3

— condemned by Peer Review Committee, 124n, 125

— damage to transplant surgery development, 125–6

surgeons,

— Ahmed, Dr Syed Adil, 147, 148

— Bailey, Leonard, 163–9, 169n

— Barnard, Professor Christiaan, 1, 57–8, 60–67, 73, 79–87, 101–3

— Calne, Sir Roy, 2–3, 40, 45, 46, 48, 128–30, 191, 204, 207–8

— Carrel, Alexis, 7–13

— Cooley, Denton, 92, 94–5, 170n

— Dubost, Charles, 29–30

— English, Sir Terence, 92n

— Fadali, Dr Moneim, 179, 203

— Hamburger, Professor Jean, 29–30, 35, 42, 49–52

— Hardy, James, 158–62

— Hitchcock, Claude, 158

— Hume, David, 29, 31–3, 58

— Iwasaki, Dr Yuji, 101n

— Kantrowitz, Adrian, 72–8, 87–8

— Kolff, Dr Wilhem, 162

— Küss, René, 29–31, 42, 44, 47, 52

— Lawler, Dr Richard H, 25–30

— Longmore, Donald, 68–70, 90

— Losman, Jacques, 167

— Lower, Richard, 96–8

— Makowka, Leonard, 170n

— McCracken, Dr Brian H., 157n

— Medawar, Sir Peter, 22–4, 39–41, 51, 120, 204

— Moore, Francis, 32, 44, 54, 89, 96

— Murray, Joseph, 33, 35, 42–4, 46, 47, 51–2

— Najarian, Dr John, 108–9, 112, 167

— Norwood, Dr William, 167n

— Patil, Dr Dilip, 147

— Reddy, Dr K.C., 143, 145–6

— Reemtsma, Keith, 156–8

— Reyes, Dr Jorge, 196, 199

— Romano, Dr Phillippe, 140

— Schlegel, Dr Jorgan, 157n

— Servelle, Marceau, 29–30

— Shumway, Dr Norman, 71–3, 88, 104

— Siddaraju, Dr K.S., 147–9

— Smith, Prentiss, 157

— Starzl, Dr Tom, 48, 53, 110, 112, 206–7

— Tchaoussoff, Dr Jean, 138–41

— Tzakis, Andreas, 192, 194, 195, 199, 201
— Wada, Professor Juro, 100
— Wallwork, John, 136, 169–70, 172–6
— White, Robert J., 180–89
— Yacoub, Magdi, 92n
survival records for transplants, 210–14
suturing of blood vessels, 13

Tannenbaum, Margo, 166, 168 *and* n
Tchaoussoff, Dr Jean, 138–41
Terasaki, Paul, 110, 111–12
Tesniere, Alain and Mireille, 138–41, 142–3
Tesniere, Christophe, 138–41
testis gland, 13–15
testosterone, 14, 18
Texas Heart Institute, Houston, 210
theft of organs for transplant, 151–3
Thiebault, Yvette, 49
Thomas, Everett, 92
Thorek, Max, 16, 18
Time magazine, 27, 157n
Times, The, 91
tissue-typing,
— avoiding immuno-suppression, 107–110
— Hague conference, 111–12
— human leukocyte antigen (HLA), 108n
— perfect match, 109n
— Terasaki theory of, 110
— *see also* skin grafts
Toronto
— General Hospital, Canada, 211
— University, Canada, 214
Transplant: The Give and Take of Tissue Transplantation (Moore), 37n, 42n
Transplantation of Tissues (Neuhof), 21n
Transplantation Proceedings, 131n

transplants,
— 'Amiens affair', 140
— animal experiments
  baboons, 158 *and* n; 162, 164–9
  cattle, skin of, 39–40
  chimpanzees, 156–61, 162n
  dogs, 10, 11, 46, 58, 70, 72, 130
  goats, 155
  mice, skin of, 40
  monkeys, 156, 182–4
  pigs, 19–21, 130, 135, 176–7, 204–5
— animals, disease problems from, 174
— cell migration in, 207–8
— cross-species, 155–6, 158, 163, 166, 168, 176–7, 204–5
— 'Holy Grail', 208
— in Japan, 100–101
— moral/ethical problems, 1, 5, 168–9, 185–6
— organs
  eyes, 138–41, 141n, 152
  heart-lungs, 132–3
  hearts *see* hearts
  kidneys *see* kidneys
  livers, 53, 54, 101n, 106–7, 196n, 196–207, 204n
  multiple organs, 2–3, 4, 63, 138, 139–40
  pancreas, 3, 5, 101n
  testes, 13–18
  whole-bodies, 6, 180–81, 183, 188
— philosophy of, 178–9, 186, 203
— and racism in America, 162
— survival records, 210–14
— waiting lists for, 5, 136
'Trojan Horse' prevention of organ rejection, 40–41, 204
Tropeano, Thomas, 200
Tsukuba University, Japan, 101n
Tucker, Bruce, 96–8
Tucker, Grover, 98
Tucker, Ruth, 25–8
Tulane University, 156

twins, kidney transplants between, 34–8
Tzakis, Andreas, 192, 194, 195, 199,
      201

UCLA *see* University College of Los
      Angeles
Ukrainian Institute of Surgery, 21
Ullman, Dr Emerich, 10n
Unger, Ernst, 20, 156n
United States Public Health Service, 34
University College of Los Angeles
      (UCLA), 108n, 110, 112
University Hospital of North Amiens,
      138–40
Ustipak, Lorraine, 108

Van Rood, Jan, 111–12
Van Zyl, Dirk, 103
vascular surgery, 10
Velu (Indian labourer), 147–51
Veterans' Administration Hospital,
      Denver, 48, 53, 110
Vetovitz, Craig, 187–8
Victoria Hospital, Bangalore, 147
Vienna University, 133n
Voronoff, Dr Sergei, 16–19
Voronoy, Yu Yu, 21, 27

Wada, Professor Juro, 100
Walker, Kenneth, 18
Wallwork, John, 136, 169–70, 172–6
Warburg Pincus (New York bank), 171
Washington Daily News, 67

Washington University, 211
Washkansky, Ann, 60, 63, 80, 84
Washkansky, Louis,
— heart patient, 56
— operation, 57–67
— post-operative problems, 79–83
   hygiene, 80
   incorrect treatment, 82
   infections, 81
   death, 83
Weppler, Nurse Debbie, 200–201
West, Fred, 90–91
White, David, 107, 128–30, 154, 171,
      172–6
White, Robert J, 6, 180–89
whole-body transplants, 6, 180–81, 183,
      188
The World of Surgery (Hardy), 162n

xenotransplantation *see* transplants,
      cross-species
X-ray radiation, 41–4, 46

Yacoub, Sir Magdi, 92n
Yelamma Desappa Hospital, India, 147,
      150
Yeoman, Paddy, 137
Yonsei University, Korea, 210

Zoology Departments of Universities,
— London, 40
— Oxford, 22
Zurich University, 214